T0226624

Arrhythmias in Athletes

Editors

DOMENICO CORRADO
CRISTINA BASSO
GAETANO THIENE

CARDIAC ELECTROPHYSIOLOGY CLINICS

www.cardiacEP.theclinics.com

Consulting Editors
RANJAN K. THAKUR
ANDREA NATALE

March 2013 • Volume 5 • Number 1

ELSEVIER

1600 John F. Kennedy Boulevard • Suite 1800 • Philadelphia, Pennsylvania, 19103-2899

http://www.theclinics.com

CARDIAC ELECTROPHYSIOLOGY CLINICS Volume 5, Number 1
March 2013 ISSN 1877-9182, ISBN-13: 978-1-4557-7067-0

Editor: Barbara Cohen-Kligerman

Cardiac Electrophysiology Clinics (ISSN 1877-9182) is published quarterly by Elsevier Inc., 360 Park Avenue South, New York, NY 10010-1710. Months of issue are March, June, September, and December. Subscription prices are $191.00 per year for US individuals, $277.00 per year for US institutions, $100.00 per year for US students and residents, $214.00 per year for Canadian individuals, $309.00 per year for Canadian institutions, $273.00 per year for international individuals, $331.00 per year for international institutions and $143.00 per year for Canadian and international students/residents. To receive student/resident rate, orders must be accompanied by name of affilliated institution, date of term, and the signature of program/residency coordinator on institution letterhead. Orders will be billed at individual rate until proof of status is received. Foreign air speed delivery is included in all Clinics subscription prices. All prices are subject to change without notice. **POSTMASTER:** Send address changes to Cardiac Electrophysiology Clinics, Elsevier Health Sciences Division, Subscription Customer Service, 3251 Riverport Lane, Maryland Heights, MO 63043. **Customer Service: 1-800-654-2452 (US and Canada). From outside of the US and Canada, call 314-477-8871. Fax: 314-447-8029. E-mail: JournalsCustomerService-usa@elsevier.com (for print support); JournalsOnlineSupport-usa@elsevier.com (for online support).**

Reprints. For copies of 100 or more of articles in this publication, please contact the Commercial Reprints Department, Elsevier Inc., 360 Park Avenue South, New York, NY 10010-1710. Tel.: 212-633-3812; Fax: 212-462-1935; E-mail: reprints@elsevier.com.

Printed and bound by CPI Group (UK) Ltd, Croydon, CR0 4YY
Transferred to Digital Printing, 2013

Contributors

CONSULTING EDITORS

RANJAN K. THAKUR, MD, MPH, MBA, FHRS
Professor of Medicine and Director, Arrhythmia Service, Thoracic and Cardiovascular Institute, Sparrow Health System, Michigan State University, Lansing, Michigan

ANDREA NATALE, MD, FACC, FHRS
Executive Medical Director, Texas Cardiac Arrhythmia Institute, St David's Medical Center, Austin, Texas; Consulting Professor, Division of Cardiology, Stanford University, Palo Alto, California; Adjunct Professor of Medicine, Heart and Vascular Center, Case Western Reserve University, Cleveland, Ohio; Director, Interventional Electrophysiology, Scripps Clinic, San Diego, California; Senior Clinical Director, EP Services, California Pacific Medical Center, San Francisco, California

EDITORS

DOMENICO CORRADO, MD, PhD
Division of Cardiology, Department of Cardiac, Thoracic and Vascular Sciences, University of Padova, Padova, Italy

CRISTINA BASSO, MD, PhD
Cardiovascular Pathology, Division of Cardiology, Department of Cardiac, Thoracic and Vascular Sciences, University of Padova, Padova, Italy

GAETANO THIENE, MD, FRCP
Cardiovascular Pathology, Division of Cardiology, Department of Cardiac, Thoracic and Vascular Sciences, University of Padova, Padova, Italy

AUTHORS

IRFAN M. ASIF, MD
Assistant Professor, Department of Family Medicine, The University of Tennessee, Knoxville, Tennessee

YOUSEF H. BADER, MD
Instructor of Medicine, The Cardiac Arrhythmia Center, Department of Medicine, Tufts Medical Center, Boston, Massachusetts

CRISTINA BASSO, MD, PhD
Cardiovascular Pathology, Division of Cardiology, Department of Cardiac, Thoracic and Vascular Sciences, University of Padova, Padova, Italy

BARBARA BAUCE, MD, PhD
Division of Cardiology, Department of Cardiac, Thoracic and Vascular Sciences, University of Padova, Padova, Italy

EMANUELE BERTAGLIA, MD
Division of Cardiology, Department of Cardiac, Thoracic and Vascular Sciences, University of Padova, Padova, Italy

FERNANDO CARDOSO BIANCHINI, MD
Division of Cardiology, Department of Cardiac, Thoracic and Vascular Sciences, University of Padova, Padova, Italy

ALESSANDRO BIFFI, MD
Department of Cardiology, Center of Sport
Medicine and Science, Rome, Italy

MATS BÖRJESSON, MD, PhD, FESC
Professor, Department of Cardiology,
Karolinska University Hospital, Solnavägen;
Swedish School of Sports and Health
Sciences, Lidingövägen, Stockholm, Sweden

CORINNA BRUNCKHORST, MD
Division of Cardiology, Cardiovascular
Centre, University Hospital Zürich, Zürich,
Switzerland

JOHN DAVID BURKHARDT, MD
Texas Cardiac Arrhythmia Institute, St. David's
Medical Center, Austin, Texas

ELISA CARTURAN, PhD
Cardiovascular Pathology, Department of
Cardiac, Thoracic and Vascular Sciences,
University of Padova, Padova, Italy

DOMENICO CORRADO, MD, PhD
Division of Cardiology, Department of Cardiac,
Thoracic and Vascular Sciences, University of
Padova, Padova, Italy

ANDERSON DONELLI DA SILVEIRA, MD
Cardiology Division, Hospital de Clínicas
de Porto Alegre, Universidade Federal do Rio
Grande do Sul, Porto Alegre, Rio Grande do
Sul, Brazil

LUIGI DI BIASE, MD, PhD
Texas Cardiac Arrhythmia Institute, St. David's
Medical Center; Department of Biomedical
Engineering, University of Texas, Austin,
Texas; Section of Electrophysiology, Albert
Einstein College of Medicine at Montefiore
Hospital, Bronx, New York; Department
of Cardiology, University of Foggia,
Foggia, Italy

JONATHAN A. DREZNER, MD
Professor, Department of Family Medicine,
University of Washington, Seattle, Washington

FIRAT DURU, MD
Division of Cardiology, Cardiovascular
Centre, University Hospital Zürich, Zürich,
Switzerland

MOHAMED ELMAGHAWRY, MD
Division of Cardiology, Department of Cardiac,
Thoracic and Vascular Sciences, University of
Padova, Padova, Italy; Department of
Cardiology, Aswan Heart Centre, Aswan,
Egypt

LAURENT HAEGELI, MD
Division of Cardiology, Cardiovascular
Centre, University Hospital Zürich, Zürich,
Switzerland

HEIN HEIDBUCHEL, MD, PhD
Department of Cardiovascular Medicine,
University Hospital Leuven, Leuven, Belgium

SABINO ILICETO, MD
Division of Cardiology, Department of Cardiac,
Thoracic and Vascular Sciences, University of
Padova, Padova, Italy

JASON JAMES, BSc
Department of Cardiovascular Sciences,
St George's University of London, London,
United Kingdom

ANDRE LA GERCHE, MBBS, PhD
Department of Cardiovascular Medicine,
University Hospital Leuven, Leuven,
Belgium; Department of Medicine,
St Vincent's Hospital, University of
Melbourne, Melbourne, Australia

LOIRA LEONI, MD, PhD
Division of Cardiology, Department of Cardiac,
Thoracic and Vascular Sciences, University of
Padova, Padova, Italy

MARK S. LINK, MD
Professor of Medicine, The Cardiac
Arrhythmia Center, Department of Medicine,
Tufts Medical School, Boston, Massachusetts

GIUSEPPE MASCIA, MD
Department of Heart and Vessels, University of
Florence, Florence, Italy

**AHMED MERGHANI, BMedSci (Hons),
MBBS, MRCP (UK)**
Department of Cardiovascular Sciences,
St George's University of London, London,
United Kingdom

FEDERICO MIGLIORE, MD
Division of Cardiology, Department of Cardiac, Thoracic and Vascular Sciences, University of Padova, Padova, Italy

ANDREA NATALE, MD, FACC, FHRS
Executive Medical Director, Texas Cardiac Arrhythmia Institute, St David's Medical Center, Austin, Texas; Consulting Professor, Division of Cardiology, Stanford University, Palo Alto, California; Adjunct Professor of Medicine, Heart and Vascular Center, Case Western Reserve University, Cleveland, Ohio; Director, Interventional Electrophysiology, Scripps Clinic, San Diego, California; Senior Clinical Director, EP Services, California Pacific Medical Center, San Francisco, California

LUIGI PADELETTI, MD
Department of Heart and Vessels, University of Florence, Florence, Italy

ANTONIO PELLICCIA, MD
Institute of Sports Medicine and Science, Rome, Italy

KALLIOPI PILICHOU, PhD
Cardiovascular Pathology, Department of Cardiac, Thoracic and Vascular Sciences, University of Padova, Padova, Italy

GEORGIANE CRESPI PONTA, MD
Division of Cardiology, Department of Cardiac, Thoracic and Vascular Sciences, University of Padova, Padova, Italy

FILIPPO M. QUATTRINI, MD, PhD
Institute of Sports Medicine and Science, Rome, Italy

ASHWIN L. RAO, MD
Assistant Professor, Department of Family Medicine, Hall Health Primary Care Center, University of Washington, Seattle, Washington

ILARIA RIGATO, MD, PhD
Division of Cardiology, Department of Cardiac, Thoracic and Vascular Sciences, University of Padova, Padova, Italy

STEFANIA RIZZO, MD
Cardiovascular Pathology, Department of Cardiac, Thoracic and Vascular Sciences, University of Padova, Padova, Italy

STEFANIA SACCHI, MD
Department of Heart and Vessels, University of Florence, Florence, Italy

PASQUALE SANTANGELI, MD
Texas Cardiac Arrhythmia Institute, St. David's Medical Center, Austin, Texas; Department of Cardiology, University of Foggia, Foggia, Italy

MAURIZIO SCHIAVON, MD
Department of Social Health, Center for Sports Medicine and Physical Activity, Padova, Italy

CHRISTIAN SCHMIED, MD
Cardiovascular Centre, University Hospital Zürich, Zürich, Switzerland

SANJAY SHARMA, MD, FRCP (UK), FESC
Professor, Department of Cardiovascular Sciences, St George's University of London, London, United Kingdom

RICARDO STEIN, ScD, MD
Cardiology Division, Hospital de Clínicas de Porto Alegre, Universidade Federal do Rio Grande do Sul, Porto Alegre, Rio Grande do Sul, Brazil

GAETANO THIENE, MD, FRCP
Cardiovascular Pathology, Division of Cardiology, Department of Cardiac, Thoracic and Vascular Sciences, University of Padova, Padova, Italy

LUC VANHEES, PhD, FESC
Full Professor, Department of Rehabilitation Sciences, Biomedical Sciences, University Leuven, Leuven, Belgium; Research Group Lifestyle and Health, Faculty of Health Care, University of Applied Sciences, Utrecht, The Netherlands

ALESSANDRO ZORZI, MD
Division of Cardiology, Department of Cardiac, Thoracic and Vascular Sciences, University of Padova, Padova, Italy

FEDERICO MIGLIORE, MD
Division of Cardiology, Department of Cardiac, Thoracic and Vascular Sciences, University of Padova, Padova, Italy

ANDREA NATALE, MD, FACC, FHRS
Executive Medical Director, Texas Cardiac Arrhythmia Institute, St. David's Medical Center, Austin, Texas; Consulting Professor, Division of Cardiology, Stanford University, Palo Alto, California; Adjunct Professor of Medicine, Heart and Vascular Center, Case Western Reserve University, Cleveland, Ohio; Director, Interventional Electrophysiology, Scripps Clinic, San Diego, California; Senior Clinical Director, EP Services, California Pacific Medical Center, San Francisco, California

LUIGI PADELETTI, MD
Department of Heart and Vessels, University of Florence, Florence, Italy

ANTONIO PELLICCIA, MD
Institute of Sports Medicine and Science, Rome, Italy

KALLIOPI PILICHOU, PhD
Cardiovascular Pathology, Department of Cardiac, Thoracic and Vascular Sciences, University of Padova, Padova, Italy

GEORGIANE CRESSI PONTA, MD
Division of Cardiology, Department of Cardiac, Thoracic and Vascular Sciences, University of Padova, Padova, Italy

FILIPPO M. QUATTRINI, MD, PhD
Institute of Sports Medicine and Science, Rome, Italy

ASHWIN L. RAO, MD
Assistant Professor, Department of Family Medicine, Hall Health Primary Care Center, University of Washington, Seattle, Washington

ILARIA RIGATO, MD, PhD
Division of Cardiology, Department of Cardiac, Thoracic and Vascular Sciences, University of Padova, Padova, Italy

STEFANIA RIZZO, MD
Cardiovascular Pathology, Department of Cardiac, Thoracic and Vascular Sciences, University of Padova, Padova, Italy

STEFANIA SACCHI, MD
Department of Heart and Vessels, University of Florence, Florence, Italy

PASQUALE SANTANGELI, MD
Texas Cardiac Arrhythmia Institute, St. David's Medical Center, Austin, Texas; Department of Cardiology, University of Foggia, Foggia, Italy

MAURIZIO SCHIAVON, MD
Department of Social Health, Center for Sports Medicine and Physical Activity, Padova, Italy

CHRISTIAN SCHMIED, MD
Cardiovascular Centre, University Hospital Zürich, Zürich, Switzerland

SANJAY SHARMA, MD, FRCP (UK), FESC
Professor, Department of Cardiovascular Sciences, St George's University of London, London, United Kingdom

RICARDO STEIN, ScD, MD
Cardiology Division, Hospital de Clínicas de Porto Alegre, Universidade Federal de Rio Grande do Sul, Porto Alegre, Rio Grande do Sul, Brazil

GAETANO THIENE, MD, FRCP
Cardiovascular Pathology, Division of Cardiology, Department of Cardiac, Thoracic and Vascular Sciences, University of Padova, Padova, Italy

LUC VANHEES, PhD, FESC
Full Professor, Department of Rehabilitation Sciences, Biomedical Sciences, University of Leuven, Leuven, Belgium; Research Group Lifestyle and Health, Faculty of Health Care, University of Applied Sciences, Utrecht, The Netherlands

ALESSANDRO ZORZI, MD
Division of Cardiology, Department of Cardiac, Thoracic and Vascular Sciences, University of Padova, Padova, Italy

Contents

Cardiovascular diseases account for 40% of all deaths in the Western countries, and nearly two-thirds of the deaths occur suddenly. Effort is a trigger with a 3-fold risk in athletes compared with nonathletes, and sports disqualification is by itself lifesaving in people with underlying concealed cardiovascular diseases. Several causes of cardiac sudden death (SD) may be identified at postmortem. The spectrum of cardiovascular substrates is wide and includes congenital and acquired diseases. In up to 20% of cases, the heart is grossly and histologically normal at autopsy. The use of molecular techniques is nowadays mandatory in cases of unexplained cardiac SD.

Competitive sports activity is associated with an increase in the risk of sudden cardiovascular death in adolescents and young adults with clinically silent cardiovascular disorders. Strategies for primary prevention include screening programs based on history and physical examination alone or including electrocardiogram (ECG). ECG screening is more sensitive and has a higher cost–benefit ratio than that based on history and physical examination alone. Modern criteria for athletes' ECG interpretation significantly improves the screening accuracy by reducing the false-positive rate (increased specificity), with the important requisite of maintaining the ability to detect life-threatening heart diseases (preserved sensitivity).

Sudden cardiac arrest (SCA) is the leading cause of death in exercising young athletes. Automated external defibrillators (AEDs) are an integral link in the "chain of survival" and their prompt use promotes higher survival rates for SCA. Public access defibrillation programs shorten the time interval between SCA and shock delivery and train likely responders in CPR and AED use. SCA should be assumed in any collapsed and unresponsive athlete. Prompt management of SCA can be life saving for athletes with SCA. This article reviews strategies for effective secondary prevention of sudden death in athletes and the critical role of AEDs.

Regular physical activity induces significant health benefits and most middle-aged/senior individuals should therefore be encouraged to increase their level of physical activity. Sporting activity may be especially beneficial because it is intense enough to increase cardiovascular, muscular, and metabolic fitness, compared with everyday physical activity. The rationale for evaluation of middle-aged/senior individuals is to ensure their safe participation in leisure-time sports, with the aim of maximizing the benefits while minimizing the risks of exercise. This article reviews the existing recommendations on evaluation of master athletes and middle-aged/senior individuals before they take part in physical activity and sports.

The reported incidence of sudden death in marathons varies widely from 0.54 to 2.1/100,000. Death in marathon runners is frequently observed in the fifth and sixth decade of life, and most deaths occur in relatively experienced runners who have participated in previous marathons. A recent study showed that runners who suffered a sudden cardiac arrest due to hypertrophic cardiomyopathy were younger and less likely to survive compared with those with coronary artery disease.

Exercise testing is an important diagnostic tool that creates an environment of automaticity at the electrical membrane, which tolerates premature beats and re-entrant arrhythmogenic circuits. Exercise testing mimics the authentic situation of physical activity and stress, recognized as a fatal trigger of critical arrhythmias in cases of underlying cardiac risk constellation. Although it is established as a second-line diagnostic tool, exercise testing can provide crucial information in an earlier setting, if there are exercise-dependent symptoms in an athlete's history, clinical suspicion of an underlying structural or primarily electrical heart disease, or known structural or electrical disease.

Several cardiomyopathies are associated with increased risk for sudden cardiac death during exercise. Physicians are required to have updated knowledge about modalities of exercise prescription relative to the type, intensity, and frequency of exercise programs that expose patients with cardiomyopathy to the lowest risk of clinical deterioration or cardiac arrest. This article offers a comprehensive overview of the current concepts governing exercise prescription and sport participation in patients with cardiomyopathies, based on the experience and insights of experts and published guidelines. The risk of sport participation in patients with cardiomyopathies is analyzed, and the main points the physician should consider in advising exercise are summarized.

Atrial fibrillation (AF) is the most common arrhythmia in the athletic community. Many studies have shown that the prevalence of AF is higher in athletes who are involved in long-term sports participation compared to the general population of the same age, and AF is more frequently observed in middle-aged than in young athletes. Sports activity may represent a facilitating factor anticipating the AF onset but does not represent the cause of AF. Catheter ablation is a particularly attractive option for athletes with AF.

Although sports participation improves quality of life and lowers cardiovascular risk, sport may represent a hazard for certain high-risk groups, such as young athletes with cardiovascular conditions necessitating an implantable cardioverter-defibrillator (ICD). There are few data weighing the risks and benefits of sports participation for patients with ICDs. Sports participants with ICDs incur the potential risk of failure of therapy, inappropriate interventions, and device injury. Severe exercise may worsen the course of the cardiovascular disease of the athlete, predisposing to more adverse clinical events. This article reviews the potential risks and recommendations for sports activity in patients with ICDs.

Erratum

An error was made in the December 2012 issue of *Cardiac Electrophysiology Clinics,* volume 4, number 4, on page 645. One of the authors of "Infra-Hisian Atrioventricular Block" was incorrectly listed as Ryan Foley. The author's correct name is T. Raymond Foley.

CARDIAC ELECTROPHYSIOLOGY CLINICS

NOW AVAILABLE FOR YOUR iPhone and iPad

Foreword
When the Best Die Young

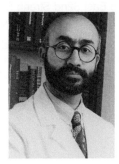
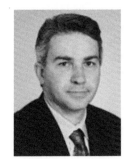

Ranjan K. Thakur, MD, MPH, MBA, FHRS   Andrea Natale, MD, FACC, FHRS
Consulting Editors

Athletes inspire us by pushing their own limits and showing what the human body is capable of achieving. For more than one hundred years, runners tried to break the 4-minute mile. It was considered the "Holy Grail" of track and field. Many said it couldn't be done. In fact, doctors wrote articles in medical journals explaining why it was physically impossible for the human body to run a mile in less than 4 minutes. On May 6th 1954, Roger Bannister, a medical student at Oxford with little training, ran a mile in 3:59.4. No sooner than "the 4-minute mile myth" was broken, 46 days later, Bannister's record was broken and since then it has been broken more than 700 times. In this way, athletes inspire us with their achievements and make it possible for others to push the limits as well. We idolize them for their physiologic achievements as well as their near-perfect physique. When an athlete dies suddenly, it leaves us bewildered as to the cause and points to our own mortality.

Until relatively recently, it was commonly thought that sudden death in athletes was due to a "heart attack" even though evidence of myocardial infarction was usually absent. The last 2 decades have revealed many causes of sudden death in younger individuals in the absence of coronary artery disease; these include coronary anomalies, hyper-

trophic cardiomyopathy, and many genetic syndromes. We have also learned much about screening tests and how to use them to prevent "the best" from dying prematurely.

This issue of the *Cardiac Electrophysiology Clinics* focuses on rhythm and conduction disturbances in athletes. Although sudden cardiac death due to ventricular arrhythmias is the ultimate feared outcome, other cardiac arrhythmias are common in athletes as well. The editors, Drs Corrado, Basso, and Thiene, are well known for their seminal contributions in this area, and they have assembled internationally renowned contributors from cardiology and sports medicine, with varied expertise.

The readers will find comprehensive, yet practical, discussions of sudden cardiac death, the role of screening and prevention, and the use of automatic external defibrillators at sporting events. Syncope, atrial arrhythmias, bradyarrhythmias, cardiomyopathies, and implantable cardioverter-defibrillators in competitive athletes are also thoroughly discussed.

This issue of the *Cardiac Electrophysiology Clinics* is of interest not only to cardiologists and electrophysiologists but also to internists, family physicians, and pediatricians, who play a critical role in the evaluation of competitive student athletes and leisure-time amateur athletes, many

Card Electrophysiol Clin 5 (2013) xiii–xiv
http://dx.doi.org/10.1016/j.ccep.2013.01.017
1877-9182/13/$ – see front matter © 2013 Published by Elsevier Inc.

of whom are quite accomplished. We hope the readership will learn much of practical use from this international panel of experts.

Ranjan K. Thakur, MD, MPH, MBA, FHRS
Sparrow Thoracic and Cardiovascular Institute
Michigan State University
1200 East Michigan Avenue; Suite 580
Lansing, MI 48912, USA

Andrea Natale, MD, FACC, FHRS
Texas Cardiac Arrhythmia Institute
Center for Atrial Fibrillation at
St. David's Medical Center
1015 East 32nd Street; Suite 516
Austin, TX 78705, USA

E-mail addresses:
thakur@msu.edu (R.K. Thakur)
andrea.natale@stdavids.com (A. Natale)

Preface

Arrhythmias in Athletes: From Pathologic Substrates to Life-Saving Shock Therapy

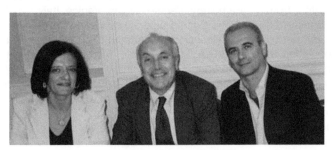

Cristina Basso, MD, PhD, Gaetano Thiene, MD, Domenico Corrado, MD, PhD
Editors

Sudden cardiac death (SCD) of an athlete is always a powerful and tragic event, which devastates families, other competitors, institutions (high school, college, or professional organization), sports medicine teams, and the community. The sudden demise of an athlete has a tremendous appeal to the media because it affects apparently healthy individuals who are regarded as heroes and the healthiest group in society. Instinctively, everyone wonders what intervention might have prevented the death. For centuries it was a mystery why cardiac arrest should occur in vigorous athletes, who had previously achieved extraordinary exercise performance without complaining of any symptoms. The cause was generally ascribed to myocardial infarction, even though evidence of ischemic myocardial necrosis was rarely reported. It is now clear that the most common mechanism of sudden death during sports activity is an abrupt arrhythmia as a consequence of a wide spectrum of cardiovascular diseases. The fact that cardiac arrest during sports activity is usually caused by abrupt ventricular fibrillation explains why demonstration of ventricular arrhythmias in the athlete is regarded as a warning sign of increased risk of SCD.

In a provocative article published in the *Lancet* in 2005, we used a quotation from the Greek dramatist Menander, "Those whom the gods love die young," in reference to SCD among athletes. We wanted to highlight that by virtue of the important results

gained by systematic investigation of SCD in young people and athletes, sports-related fatalities should no longer be considered as predestined and beyond our control, but a consequence of an underlying heart disease that may be identified and treated during life.

An international panel of cardiologists and sports medical physicians, with expertise in the fields of cardiovascular pathology, electrophysiology, athletic screening, and management of athletes, has contributed to this issue of *Cardiac Electrophysiology Clinics*, which is designed to offer a comprehensive overview of rhythm and conduction distubances in athletes and will be an essential reference for clinical cardiologists, sports medicine doctors, and general practitioners on early diagnosis, risk stratification, and therapy for arrhythmic events with the aim of preventing sports-related SCD.

The issue first addresses the etiopathogenesis of SCD in the athlete and its prevention by either preparticipation screening (primary prevention) or the use of an automated external defibrillator in the field (secondary prevention). The vast majority of athletes who die suddenly have underlying structural heart diseases, which provide a substrate for ventricular tachycardia/fibrillation leading to cardiac arrest. There is compelling evidence that timely recognition by electrocardiographic screening of cardiovascular diseases that

Card Electrophysiol Clin 5 (2013) xv–xvi
http://dx.doi.org/10.1016/j.ccep.2013.01.016
1877-9182/13/$ – see front matter © 2013 Published by Elsevier Inc.

pose a risk of life-threatening arrhythmias in the athlete is life-saving. A time-trend analysis of the incidence of SCD in young competitive athletes aged between 12 and 35 years in the Veneto region of Italy between 1979 and 2004 demonstrated a sharp decline of approximately 90% in death rates among athletes after the introduction of the national screening program in 1982, particularly because of fewer sudden deaths from cardiomyopathies. By comparison, mortality did not change significantly over the study period among the unscreened sedentary population. A parallel study of a large population of young competitive athletes undergoing preparticipation screening at the Centre for Sports Medicine showed that the decline in mortality from cardiomyopathies paralleled the concomitant increase in the number of affected athletes who were identified and disqualified from competitive sports over the screening period. Automated external defibrillators (AEDs) are an integral link in the "chain of survival" and their prompt use promotes higher survival rates from sudden cardiac arrest during sports. The presence of a free-standing AED at sporting events is a valuable backup for unpredictable arrhythmic cardiac arrest due to conditions unrecognized by electrocardiographic screening.

This *Cardiac Electrophysiology Clinics* issue provides considerable information on the cardiovascular evaluation of leisure-time master athletes and marathon runners, on the role of exercise testing for risk stratification, and on specific problems with treatment of athletes presenting with syncope, atrial fibrillation, or bradyarrhythmias. The topic of heart muscle disease and sports is also covered, with particular reference to a possible exercise-induced right ventricular cardiomyopathy in overtrained athletes. Finally, there is a discussion on the safety and arrhythmic risks of sports activity in those with an internal implantable defibrillator.

We are confident that the issue will help physicians in the complex management of arrhythmias occurring in individuals engaged in sports activity, which represents a frequent clinical challenge because of the increased sports participation at all ages.

ACKNOWLEDGMENTS

The Editors and their groups are supported by the Fondazione Cariparo, Padova and Rovigo; and by the Registry of Cardio-Cerebro-Vascular Pathology, Veneto Region, Venice, Italy.

The Editors also acknowledge the Association for Research of Arrhythmic Cardiac Diseases (A.R.C.A., via Gabelli, 61, 35121 Padua-Italy; http://anpat.unipd.it/arca/) and Mrs Chiara Carturan and Mr Marco Pizzigolotto for their assistance in preparing this book.

Domenico Corrado, MD, PhD
Division of Cardiology
Department of Cardiac, Thoracic and
Vascular Sciences
University of Padova
Via Giustiniani, 2
35121 Padova, Italy

Cristina Basso, MD, PhD
Cardiovascular Pathology
Department of Cardiac, Thoracic and
Vascular Sciences
University of Padova
Via A. Gabelli 61
35121 Padova, Italy

Gaetano Thiene, MD
Cardiovascular Pathology
Department of Cardiac, Thoracic and
Vascular Sciences
University of Padova
Via A. Gabelli 61
35121 Padova, Italy

E-mail addresses:
domenico.corrado@unipd.it (D. Corrado)
cristina.basso@unipd.it (C. Basso)
gaetano.thiene@unipd.it (G. Thiene)

Pathologic Substrates of Sudden Cardiac Death During Sports

Cristina Basso, MD, PhD[a],*, Elisa Carturan, PhD[a],
Kalliopi Pilichou, PhD[a], Stefania Rizzo, MD[a],
Domenico Corrado, MD, PhD[b], Gaetano Thiene, MD[a]

KEYWORDS

- Autopsy • Cardiomyopathies • Coronary artery disease • Pathologic substrates • Sport activity
- Sudden death

KEY POINTS

- Several culprits of cardiac sudden death (SD) may be identified at postmortem; atherosclerotic coronary artery disease (CAD) is the leading cause (25% of SD cases in the young), mostly consisting of a single obstructive plaque with fibrocellular intimal proliferation.
- The spectrum of cardiovascular substrates is wide and also includes congenital diseases of the coronary arteries (mainly anomalous origin), myocardium (arrhythmogenic and hypertrophic cardiomyopathies, myocarditis), valves (aortic stenosis and mitral valve prolapse), and conduction system (ventricular preexcitation, accelerated atrioventricular (AV) conduction and AV block).
- In up to 20% of cases, the heart is grossly and histologically normal at autopsy (unexplained SD or "mors sine materia"); in such cases, inherited ion channel diseases have been implicated (long and short QT syndromes, Brugada syndrome, and catecholaminergic polymorphic ventricular tachycardia).
- Use of molecular techniques at autopsy is nowadays mandatory in cases of unexplained cardiac SD.
- Doping and other substances of abuse should always be excluded by rigorous methodology and use of standardized protocols.

INTRODUCTION

Sudden death (SD) in the young and in the athlete is mostly cardiovascular in origin; cerebral or respiratory causes are rare.[1–5] Sport activity is a double-edged sword; although it offers protection from the risk of SD in those people who regularly engage in exercise, it can increase the short-term risk of SD due to underlying, frequently concealed heart disease. In a previous study of incidence of SD in the young and in the athletes (≤35 years), performed in 300 young people who died suddenly in the northeast of Italy, the authors calculated a cumulative rate of 1 per 100,000 per year.[4] Surprisingly, the rate of cardiovascular SD was nearly 3-fold in athletes when compared with nonathletes (2.3 to 0.9). The added risk was particularly high in subjects who were unaware of being affected by congenital anomalies of coronary arteries (relative risk = 79), arrhythmogenic right ventricular cardiomyopathy (ARVC) (relative

Disclosures: No conflicts of interest to declare.
Sources of funding: This study was supported by the CARIPARO Foundation, Padua, Italy, and the Registry for Cardio-cerebro-vascular Pathology, Veneto Region, Venice, Italy.
[a] Cardiovascular Pathology, Department of Cardiac, Thoracic and Vascular Sciences, University of Padova, Via A. Gabelli 61, 35121, Padova, Italy; [b] Division of Cardiology, Department of Cardiac, Thoracic and Vascular Sciences, University of Padova, Via Giustiniani 2, 35120, Padova, Italy
* Corresponding author. Cardiovascular Pathology, Department of Cardiac, Thoracic and Vascular Sciences, University of Padova, Via A. Gabelli 61, 35121, Padova, Italy.
E-mail address: cristina.basso@unipd.it

Card Electrophysiol Clin 5 (2013) 1–11
http://dx.doi.org/10.1016/j.ccep.2013.01.002
1877-9182/13/$ – see front matter © 2013 Elsevier Inc. All rights reserved.

risk = 5.4) and atherosclerotic coronary artery disease (CAD) (relative risk = 2.6).[4,5]

Pathologists are responsible for determining the precise cause of SD, but there is considerable variation in the way in which they approach this complex task. The Association for European Cardiovascular Pathology (AECVP) developed guidelines that represent the minimum standard that is required in the routine autopsy practice for the adequate assessment of cardiac SD, including a protocol not only for heart examination and histologic sampling but also for toxicology and molecular investigation.[6] As stressed in the AECVP guidelines, the postmortem report should conclude with a clear clinico-pathologic summary (epicrisis). In most SDs, a clear pathologic cause can be identified, albeit with varying degrees of confidence. Wherever possible, the most likely underlying cause should be stated and the need for familial clinical screening and genetic analysis clearly indicated.

From the physiopathology viewpoint, cardiovascular SD can be either "mechanical" or "electric". In the former, heart function is impaired by an acute blockage of the blood circulation (pulmonary embolism) or by cardiac tamponade (hemopericardium due to heart or aortic rupture). Shock due to massive hemorrhage (extrapericardial aortic rupture, gastrointestinal bleeding) or due to adrenal septic apoplexy may also be considered a mechanical SD.[1-3]

Aortic rupture in the young is mostly associated with congenital or inherited diseases, such as bicuspid aortic valve with or without isthmic coarctation, and Marfan syndrome.[7] In Marfan syndrome, the risk is nowadays easily predictable and surgery indicated when the diameter of the ascending aorta exceeds 5 cm, whereas the bicuspid aortic valve is mostly concealed and rupture of the aorta may represent the first manifestation of the disease.[8] Moreover, in Marfan syndrome the molecular defect has been found mostly in mutations of the fibrillin gene, whereas in the bicuspid valve the defect is still unknown. The bicuspid aortic valve is a frequent disorder, with an incidence of 0.5%–1% in the general population[8] and may be hereditary. When diagnosed, echo monitoring is mandatory to follow up either ascending aorta diameters or elasticity.[9,10]

However, in more than 90% of SD cases the mechanism of cardiac arrest is arrhythmic (electric), with an acute pump failure due to asystole or ventricular fibrillation.[1-3] The latter, which is by far the most frequent mechanism, should not necessarily be considered lethal because there are rescue measurements available (external or implantable defibrillator), which, by promptly delivering an electric shock, may reverse fibrillation into regular sinus rhythm.

CARDIAC DISEASE AT RISK OF ARRHYTHMIC SUDDEN DEATH IN THE YOUNG

Arrhythmic cardiac SD has several causes, that is, diseases of the coronary arteries, the myocardium, the valves, and the conduction system.[1-3]

The variable study design, more than geographic or ethnic reasons, can explain the differences in the prevalence of cardiovascular substrates of SD in the several series available in the literature. Since 1979, the Italian study has relied on systematic investigation according to a prospective study design and the collection of juvenile SDs occurring in the Veneto region, with morphologic examination of all hearts performed by the same team of experienced cardiovascular pathologists according to a standard protocol.[11] This explains also the low proportion of cases with a clear diagnosis of the cause of SD (only 24.7%) in the French series by Marijon and colleagues,[12] in which the autopsy was available only in a small subgroup of cases. Moreover, the United States cardiac SD rates reported by Maron and colleagues[13] were based mostly on a retrospective analysis of data provided by different sources such as news media, the Web, and others. **Fig. 1** reports the causes of cardiac SD in the athletes in 2 different series from the United States and Italy.

Atherosclerotic CAD

A single obstructive plaque located in the proximal left anterior descending coronary artery may be enough for triggering ventricular fibrillation and SD.[14] Coronary thrombosis is much less frequent than SD in adults, and it is due more to endothelial erosion than to plaque rupture (**Fig. 2A**).

Vasospasm, superimposed on a single obstructive plaque, seems to play a major role as a precipitating mechanism leading to transient coronary occlusion, with lethal ventricular fibrillation triggered by reperfusion at the time of coronary artery reopening. The intriguing aspect is that ischemia is recorded neither at the basal 12-lead electrocardiography (ECG) nor following a stress test, so that athletes, for instance, may escape the preparticipation screening, which includes ECG.[15] Use of noninvasive imaging of the coronary artery tree by magnetic resonance or computed tomography might help to identify subjects at risk.

Congenital Anomalies of Coronary Arteries

Anomalous origin of a coronary artery from the pulmonary trunk is considered a major malformation

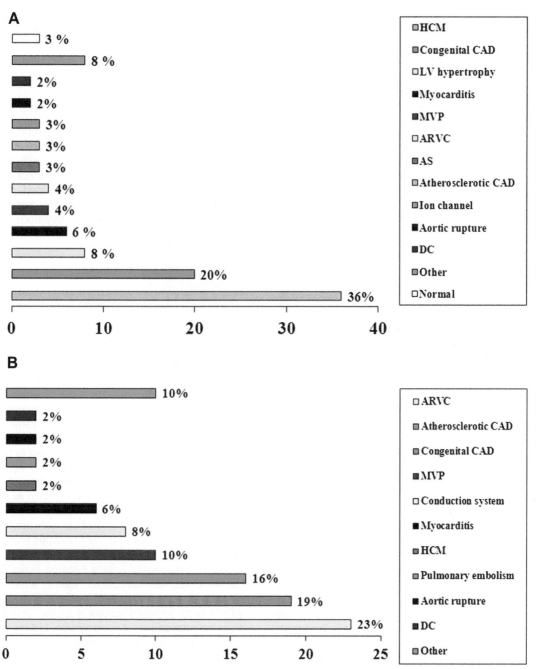

Fig. 1. Cardiovascular causes of sudden death in the athletes: the United States (*A*) versus Italy (*B*) series. ARVC, arrhythmogenic right ventricular cardiomyopathy; AS, aortic stenosis; CAD, coronary artery disease; DC, dilated cardiomyopathy; HCM, hypertrophic cardiomyopathy; LV, left ventricle; MVP, mitral valve prolapse. (*Data from* Maron BJ. Hypertrophic cardiomyopathy and other causes of sudden cardiac death in young competitive athletes, with considerations for preparticipation screening and criteria for disqualification. Cardiol Clin 2007;25:399–414; and Corrado D, Basso C, Rizzoli G, et al. Does sports activity enhance the risk of sudden death in adolescents and young adults? J Am Coll Cardiol 2003;42:1959–63.)

in so far as, after birth, a steal of blood occurs from the aorta to the pulmonary artery via the coronary arterial system, causing severe myocardial damage.[16–19] However, it is usually a highly symptomatic disease since infancy, and it is exceptionally observed in young athletes.

There are apparently minor coronary artery malformations, which are life threatening during effort.

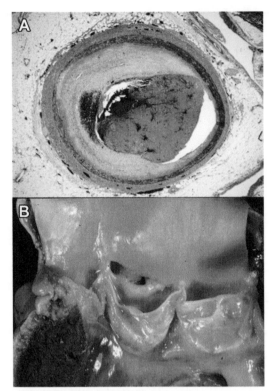

Fig. 2. Sudden death by coronary artery disease. (*A*) Atherosclerosis with thrombosis due to endothelial erosion. (*B*) Anomalous origin of the left coronary artery from the right aortic sinus of Valsalva. Note the absence of a coronary ostium in the left coronary sinus and the presence of 2 ostia in the right coronary sinus (sudden death during jogging).

This is the case of the anomalous origin of a coronary artery from the opposite sinus of Valsalva: left coronary artery from the right coronary sinus or right coronary artery from the left coronary sinus.[17–19] Although both coronary arteries originate from the aorta, the coronary artery with anomalous origin presents with an acute angle take-off and an intramural aortic course, with an interarterial course behind the pulmonary artery and a slit-like lumen (see **Fig. 2**B), all conditions predisposing to impaired coronary blood flow during effort. Repetitive myocardial ischemic damage occurs during strenuous exercise, with reperfusion injury followed by fibrotic repair, all prerequisites for the onset of ominous ventricular arrhythmias and even ventricular fibrillation.[19] Anomalous origin of the left coronary artery from the right sinus is the worst condition because the large anteroseptal ventricular myocardium is at risk. Again, the basal and step test ECG may be normal, and the malformation may escape the preparticipation screening. In the presence of symptoms, particularly during effort, such as angina, syncopal episodes, or palpitation,

exploration of the aortic root by noninvasive imaging such as 2-dimensional (2D) echo, magnetic resonance, or computed tomography may be of great help in detecting the anomaly.[19] Sport disqualification with avoidance of strenuous exercise is lifesaving.

Other apparently benign coronary artery anomalies may rarely be lethal during effort[17] and include the anomalous origin of the left circumflex coronary artery from right sinus or from right coronary artery, with retroaortic course[20]; the deep intramyocardial course of the left anterior descending coronary artery, often associated with hypertrophic cardiomyopathy (HCM)[21,22]; and the high take-off of a major coronary artery from the tubular portion of the ascending aorta.[17]

Arrhythmogenic Right Ventricular Cardiomyopathy

According to the experience from the Veneto Region, northeast of Italy, ARVC is the second cause of SD in the young[2,23,24] and ranks first among the athletes.[4,15] The disease is characterized by life-threatening ventricular arrhythmias of right ventricular origin, with left bundle branch block morphology, as a consequence of the progressive myocardial atrophy with cardiomyocyte death and fibrofatty replacement (**Fig. 3**).[23,24] Aneurysms in the inflow, apex, and outflow right ventricular free wall (triangle of dysplasia) can be detected in the overt forms, in the absence of CAD.[24–26] Apart from ventricular arrhythmias, there are subtle ECG abnormalities that are pathognomonic, such as inverted T waves in right precordial leads, enlarged QRS (>110 ms), and late potentials with epsilon wave.[27] Inverted T waves may be an isolated finding in the absence of morphofunctional abnormalities at echo.[28,29] Diagnostic criteria became available as to make diagnosis feasible and identify affected patients and have been recently updated.[30]

ARVC is an inherited cardiomyopathy, usually with autosomal dominant transmission, but recessive forms associated with palmoplantar keratosis and woolly hair, as in the cardiocutaneous syndromes, have also been described.[25,26] The relationship between skin and cardiac involvement was explained through molecular investigations that were able to detect mutations of genes encoding defective proteins of the desmosome, a cell junction structure present in both the cardiomyocytes and epidermal cells.

Electroanatomic mapping of the right ventricular free wall increases the diagnostic accuracy and is useful in indicating areas for performing endomyocardial biopsy and radiofrequency ablation.[31,32] Advances in diagnosis were obtained with the

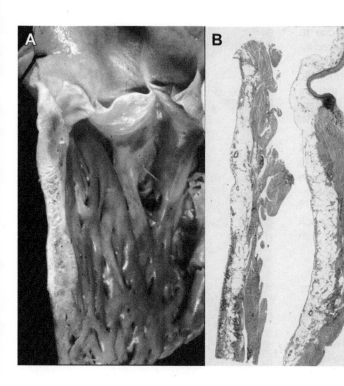

Fig. 3. Sudden death in a soccer player during effort due to arrhythmogenic right ventricular cardiomyopathy. (*A*) Gross view of the right ventricular outflow tract showing transmural myocardial atrophy with fibrofatty replacement; (*B*) corresponding panoramic histologic sections.

use of cardiac magnetic resonance with late enhancement (gadolinium), especially when the left ventricle is involved.[33]

Hypertrophic Cardiomyopathy

This condition is reported as the major cause of SD in athletes in the United States, in up to 40% of cases.[13,34] Geographic and ethnic reasons may explain the different rates of ARVC and HCM in Europe and the United States. Basal 12-lead ECG presents with abnormalities (increased QRS voltage, inverted T wave in left precordial leads, and Q waves).[35] Although these ECG abnormalities are nonspecific, they render compulsory the use of 2D echo, according to the Italian preparticipation screening protocol for sports eligibility,[36] thus making diagnosis easy.[15,35]

HCM is hereditary with autosomal dominant transmission and was found through molecular studies to be mostly a disease of the sarcomere, due to mutations of genes coding proteins of the contractile apparatus (β myosin heavy chain, myosin binding protein C, tropomyosin, and troponins).[37]

The disease is featured by asymmetric left ventricular hypertrophy, usually anteroseptal (**Fig. 4**) and rarely apical, not explained by left ventricular pressure overload. HCM is highly arrhythmogenic, and SD is the usual mode of fatal outcome.[22,38] Arrhythmic substrates reside in the cardiac hypertrophy, myocardial disarray, and scarring of the

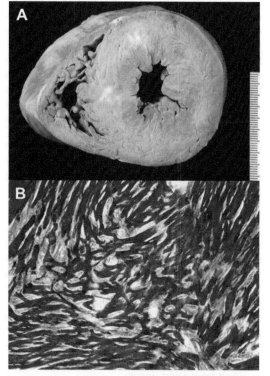

Fig. 4. Sudden death in a cyclist during effort due to hypertrophic cardiomyopathy. (*A*) Gross view of the heart, cross section. Note the severe concentric asymmetric hypertrophy with septal scars. (*B*) At histology, diffuse myocardial fibers disarray with interstitial fibrosis.

myocardium, following ischemic damage due to small arteries compression because of increased intramyocardial diastolic pressure and hypertrophy with impaired coronary reserve.[38] In a morphologic analysis of more than 250 hearts, the authors demonstrated that myocardial bridge is a frequent component of phenotypically expressed HCM. Although no systematic association with HCM-related SD was evident, their findings did not exclude the possibility that this coronary artery anomaly could contribute to increased risk in some individual patients, potentially affecting management decision making on a case-by-case basis.[22] Scars are detectable by noninvasive imaging such as late enhancement magnetic resonance with gadolinium.

Myocarditis

Myocarditis, also known as inflammatory cardiomyopathy, is a cause of SD in nearly 10% of young people.[2,3,39] It is usually infective in origin, mostly due to RNA and DNA cardiotropic viruses such as enterovirus or adenovirus, which may involve the myocardium in the setting of gastroenteric or respiratory infections.[39] Even focal myocarditis, with preserved pump function, may be life-threatening by triggering ventricular arrhythmias. Etiologic diagnosis may be achieved in vivo by endomyocardial biopsy or even at postmortem, using molecular biological techniques (**Fig. 5**). Effort is a major trigger in precipitating arrhythmias and should be avoided during the acute phase of myocarditis until the disease has completely resolved. Athletes should be temporarily excluded from competitive and amateur leisure time sport activity regardless of age, gender, severity of symptoms, and therapeutic regimen. After resolution of the clinical presentation (at least 6 months after the onset of the disease), clinical reassessment is indicated before the athlete resumes competitive sport.[40]

Valve diseases

Arrhythmic SD may occur in the setting of aortic stenosis and mitral valve prolapse.[1–3] Congenital aortic stenosis, due to either bicuspid or unicuspid valve, is an arrhythmogenic disorder in so far as left ventricular hypertrophy due to a stenotic aortic orifice with systolic overload determines subendocardial ischemia, necrosis, and scarring, which are aggravated by repetitive, prolonged efforts.[41] Because of systolic murmur, affected patients are easily detectable by 2D echo and thus disqualified from sport activity.

Mitral valve prolapse affects mainly young women and may be silent in the absence of valve incompetence.[42] Subjects may present with polymorphic ventricular arrhythmias. The

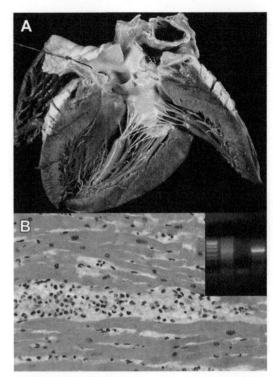

Fig. 5. Sudden death due to viral myocarditis. (*A*) The heart is grossly normal. (*B*) Histology shows inflammatory infiltrates in the myocardium; in the inset, molecular biological investigation of the myocardium reveals enteroviral infection (lane 1, size maker; lane 2, sudden death case; lane 3, enterovirus control negative; lane 4, enterovirus control positive).

arrhythmic substrate often consists of spots of replacement-type fibrosis and increased extracellular matrix, as occurring in the mitral valve leaflets themselves. Clearly, effort may aggravate the risk of life-threatening arrhythmias.

Conduction system disorders

Abnormalities of the conduction system, both congenital and acquired, may underlie SD.[1–3] Ventricular preexcitation, most frequently in the form of Wolff-Parkinson-White (WPW) syndrome, with accessory atrio-ventricular (AV) fascicle bypassing the specialized AV junction outside the regular AV conduction system,[43,44] may be also at high risk. Since the accessory pathway consists of working myocardium lacking decremental properties, an episode of atrial fibrillation may transform into ventricular fibrillation with 1 to 1 AV conduction of the electrical impulse.[44]

In the Italian experience, WPW syndrome was a rare cause of SD in athletes, because short PQ interval with delta wave was usually observed at ECG during preparticipation screening; it was then possible to ablate the aberrant fascicle, thus interrupting the anomalous AV connection, which is the pathway of arrhythmias.

Acquired AV block (Lenègre disease), consisting of progressive fibrosis of the specialized AV junction (especially bifurcating the His bundle and bundle branches), may be hidden and manifest with apparently benign bundle branch block.[45] The onset of AV block may be sudden and fatal.

The inherited variant is due to mutations of the sodium channel (SCN5A) and may overlap with the Brugada syndrome, which is also frequently characterized by a prolonged PQ interval and right bundle branch block, besides ST segment elevation.[46]

Sudden cardiac death with structurally normal heart

There are cardiac SD cases in which the heart appears structurally normal, at gross, histologic, and ultrastructural investigations (mors sine materia or unexplained SD).[1–3,47,48] They represent 10%–20% of all juvenile SDs and are due to inherited cardiomyopathies with isolated electric dysfunction, due to defective proteins of sodium and potassium ion channels at the sarcolemma level or receptors for intracellular calcium release.[48,49]

Long QT syndrome, in both autosomal and recessive forms, is characterized by prolonged QT interval, mostly due to potassium channel dysfunction in terms of delay of intracellular potassium current during repolarization.[50] On the opposite, in short QT syndrome, a hereditary disease with autosomal dominant transmission, the potassium reentry is accelerated during repolarization.[51] Both conditions are at risk of SD: the more the length or shortness of the QT interval, respectively, the higher the risk of ventricular fibrillation.

Brugada[52] or Martini-Nava-Thiene[53] syndrome is an inherited autosomal dominant cardiomyopathy, featured by nonischemic ST segment elevation, due to delayed sodium exit during repolarization. Whether there are structural alterations associated with Brugada syndrome is still a matter of controversy.[54]

All the above-mentioned arrhythmic disorders present with abnormalities at the basal ECG. As such, they should be easily diagnosed or suspected. On the opposite, catecholaminergic polymorphic ventricular tachycardia presents with normal ECG at rest; ventricular arrhythmias arise only during effort or emotion, when the heart frequency exceeds the threshold of 120–130 beats/min. It is also an inherited disease with an autosomal dominant pattern. Molecular investigations disclosed mutations in genes coding the calcium receptors (ryanodine receptor 2 and calsequestrin) located in the membrane of the smooth sarcoplasmic reticulum and in charge of calcium release for electromechanical coupling.[55,56]

Unfortunately, the stress test result may be false negative, so that only genetic screening may detect asymptomatic carriers and allow preventive strategies.[57] Autopsy may still represent the first opportunity to make the proper diagnosis, and the use of molecular biological techniques even at postmortem may be of help in solving the puzzle of mors sine materia.[1–3,6,48]

However, molecular autopsy, performed in a large cohort of cases, was able to achieve the diagnosis in only 34% of unexplained SD cases (14% RyR2, 16% KCNQ1 or KCNH2, and 4% SCN5A), whereas the remaining cases were negative,[49] which means that the cause of two-thirds of mors sine materia is still unknown.

The use of molecular techniques at autopsy is nowadays mandatory in cases of unexplained cardiac SD and has been recommended in the guidelines for autopsy investigation proposed by the AECVP.[6,48,58]

Doping Substances in Athletes

Athletes use anabolic-androgenic steroids to increase strength and lean body mass and, in some cases, to improve physical appearance.[59] The lifetime prevalence of anabolic-androgenic steroids use among adolescent boys in Western countries typically ranges from 1% to 5%.[60] According to the International Olympic Committee, steroids account for more than 50% of doping cases with positive results.[61] Although the topic is still being debated and most of the evidence is anecdotal, a consensus is beginning to emerge that chronic anabolic-androgenic steroids abuse may be associated with an increased risk of SD, myocardial infarction, altered serum lipoprotein levels, and cardiac hypertrophy. The authors reported 4 cases of SD of previously healthy athletes who were anabolic-androgenic steroid users.[59] Concentric cardiac hypertrophy with focal fibrosis, dilated cardiomyopathy with patchy myocyte death, and eosinophilic myocarditis were observed and most probably relate to the final event (**Fig. 6**).

Furthermore, in southeast of Spain, systematic toxicology investigation indicates that 3.1% of SDs are cocaine related and are mainly due to cardiocerebrovascular causes. Left ventricular hypertrophy, small vessel disease, and premature atherosclerotic CAD, with or without lumen thrombosis, are frequent findings that may account for

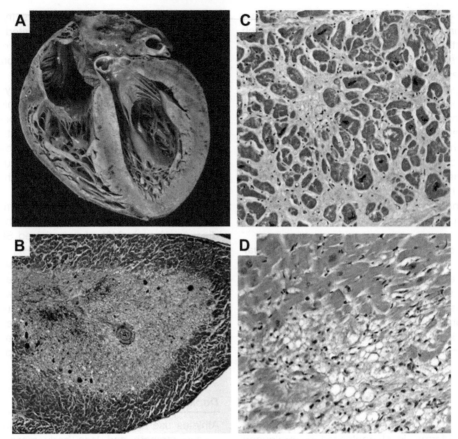

Fig. 6. Sudden death in an anabolic steroid abuser. Note the eccentric biventricular hypertrophy with chamber dilatation (*A*), myocytolysis in the subendocardial trabeculae (*B*), hypertrophic myocytes with dysmetric and dysmorphic nuclei (*C*), and myocyte vacuolization with rare inflammatory infiltrates (*D*).

myocardial ischemia at risk of cardiac arrest in persons addicted to cocaine.[62]

It must be emphasized that the cause–effect relationship between drug abuse and SD can be established only by rigorous methodology and use of standardized protocols, including precise morphologic studies of all target organs, to search for chronic toxic effects (morphologic indicators for consumption). Laboratory investigations should be aimed at searching for abuse drugs on a wide range of biologic matrices to demonstrate type, magnitude, and time of exposure. The diagnosis of doping-related SD in athletes is another paradigmatic example of the need for an integrated methodological approach based on the evaluation of clinicoanamnestic data, pathologic findings (macroscopic and microscopic), and laboratory (chemical, toxicologic, and molecular) data.[6]

SUMMARY

Cardiovascular diseases account for 40% of all deaths in the Western countries, and nearly two-thirds of them occur suddenly. Effort is a trigger of SD with a 3-fold risk in athletes compared with nonathletes, and sports disqualification is by itself lifesaving in people with underlying concealed cardiovascular diseases. Several causes of cardiac SD may be identified at postmortem, and atherosclerotic CAD is the leading cause (25% of SD cases in the young), mostly consisting of a single obstructive plaque. However, the spectrum of cardiovascular substrates is wide and includes also congenital diseases of the coronary arteries (mainly anomalous origin), myocardium (arrhythmogenic and hypertrophic cardiomyopathies, myocarditis), valves (aortic stenosis and mitral valve prolapse), and conduction system. In up to 20% of cases, the heart is grossly and histologically normal at autopsy (unexplained SD or mors sine materia), and inherited ion channel diseases have been implicated (long and short QT syndromes, Brugada syndrome, and catecholaminergic polymorphic ventricular tachycardia). The use of molecular techniques at autopsy is nowadays mandatory in cases of unexplained cardiac SD. Finally, doping and other substances of abuse should be always excluded by rigorous methodology and use of standardized protocols.

REFERENCES

1. Thiene G, Basso C, Corrado D. Cardiovascular causes of sudden death. In: Silver MD, Gotlieb AI, Schoen FJ, editors. Cardiovascular pathology. 3rd edition. Philadelphia: Churchill Livingstone; 2001. p. 326–74.
2. Basso C, Calabrese F, Corrado D, et al. Postmortem diagnosis in sudden cardiac death victims: macroscopic, microscopic and molecular findings. Cardiovasc Res 2001;50:290–300.
3. Thiene G, Carturan E, Corrado D, et al. Prevention of sudden cardiac death in the young and in athletes: dream or reality? Cardiovasc Pathol 2010;19:207–17.
4. Corrado D, Basso C, Rizzoli G, et al. Does sports activity enhance the risk of sudden death in adolescents and young adults? J Am Coll Cardiol 2003;42: 1959–63.
5. Thiene G, Corrado D, Rigato I, et al. Why and how to support screening strategies to prevent sudden death in athletes. Cell Tissue Res 2012;348:315–8.
6. Basso C, Burke M, Fornes P, et al, Association for European Cardiovascular Pathology. Guidelines for autopsy investigation of sudden cardiac death. Virchows Arch 2008;452:11–8.
7. Basso C, Frescura C, Corrado D, et al. Congenital heart disease and sudden death in the young. Hum Pathol 1995;26:1065–72.
8. Basso C, Boschello M, Perrone C, et al. An echo-cardiographic survey of primary school children for bicuspid aortic valve. Am J Cardiol 2004;93: 661–3.
9. Nistri S, Sorbo MD, Marin M, et al. Aortic root dilatation in young men with normally functioning bicuspid aortic valves. Heart 1999;82:19–22.
10. Nistri S, Grande-Allen J, Noale M, et al. Aortic elasticity and size in bicuspid aortic valve syndrome. Eur Heart J 2008;29:472–9.
11. Corrado D, Basso C, Thiene G. Comparison of United States and Italian experiences with sudden cardiac deaths in young competitive athletes: are the athletic populations comparable? Am J Cardiol 2010;105:421–2.
12. Marijon E, Tafflet M, Celermajer DS, et al. Sports-related sudden death in the general population. Circulation 2011;124:672–81.
13. Maron BJ. Hypertrophic cardiomyopathy and other causes of sudden cardiac death in young competitive athletes, with considerations for preparticipation screening and criteria for disqualification. Cardiol Clin 2007;25:399–414.
14. Corrado D, Basso C, Poletti A, et al. Sudden death in the young: is coronary thrombosis the major precipitating factor? Circulation 1994;90:2315–23.
15. Corrado D, Basso C, Pavei A, et al. Trends in sudden cardiovascular death in young competitive athletes after implementation of a preparticipation screening program. JAMA 2006;296:1593–601.
16. Thiene G, Basso C. Sudden coronary death–not always atherosclerotic. Heart 2010;96:1084–5.
17. Frescura C, Basso C, Thiene G, et al. Anomalous origin of coronary arteries and risk of sudden death: a study based on an autopsy population of congenital heart disease. Hum Pathol 1998;29:689–95.
18. Corrado D, Thiene G, Cocco P, et al. Non-atherosclerotic coronary artery disease and sudden death in the young. Br Heart J 1992;68:601–7.
19. Basso C, Maron BJ, Corrado D, et al. Clinical profile of congenital coronary artery anomalies with origin from the wrong aortic sinus leading to sudden death in young competitive athletes. J Am Coll Cardiol 2000;35:1493–501.
20. Corrado D, Pennelli T, Piovesana PG, et al. Anomalous origin of the left circumflex coronary artery from the right aortic sinus of Valsalva and sudden death. Cardiovasc Pathol 1994;3:269–71.
21. Gori F, Basso C, Thiene G. Myocardial infarction in a patient with hypertrophic cardiomyopathy. N Engl J Med 2000;342:593–4.
22. Basso C, Thiene G, Mackey-Bojack S, et al. Myocardial bridging, a frequent component of the hypertrophic cardiomyopathy phenotype, lacks systematic association with sudden cardiac death. Eur Heart J 2009;30:1627–34.
23. Thiene G, Nava A, Corrado D, et al. Right ventricular cardiomyopathy and sudden death in young people. N Engl J Med 1988;318:129–33.
24. Basso C, Thiene G, Corrado D, et al. Arrhythmogenic right ventricular cardiomyopathy: dysplasia, dystrophy, or myocarditis? Circulation 1996;94: 983–91.
25. Basso C, Bauce B, Corrado D, et al. Pathophysiology of arrhythmogenic cardiomyopathy. Nat Rev Cardiol 2011;9:223–33.
26. Basso C, Corrado D, Bauce B, et al. Arrhythmogenic right ventricular cardiomyopathy. Circ Arrhythm Electrophysiol 2012;5:1233–46.
27. Basso C, Corrado D, Marcus FI, et al. Arrhythmogenic right ventricular cardiomyopathy. Lancet 2009;373:1289–300.
28. Pelliccia A, Di Paolo FM, Quattrini FM, et al. Outcomes in athletes with marked ECG repolarization abnormalities. N Engl J Med 2008;358: 152–61.
29. Migliore F, Zorzi A, Michieli P, et al. Prevalence of cardiomyopathy in Italian asymptomatic children with electrocardiographic T-wave inversion at preparticipation screening. Circulation 2012;125:529–38.

30. Marcus FI, McKenna WJ, Sherrill D, et al. Diagnosis of arrhythmogenic right ventricular cardiomyopathy/dysplasia: proposed modification of the task force criteria. Circulation 2010;121:1533–41.

31. Corrado D, Basso C, Leoni L, et al. Three-dimensional electroanatomic voltage mapping increases accuracy of diagnosing arrhythmogenic right ventricular cardiomyopathy/dysplasia. Circulation 2005;111:3042–50.

32. Basso C, Ronco F, Marcus F, et al. Quantitative assessment of endomyocardial biopsy in arrhythmogenic right ventricular cardiomyopathy/displasia: an in vitro validation of diagnostic criteria. Eur Heart J 2008;29:2760–71.

33. Marra MP, Leoni L, Bauce B, et al. Imaging study of ventricular scar in arrhythmogenic right ventricular cardiomyopathy: comparison of 3D standard electroanatomical voltage mapping and contrast-enhanced cardiac magnetic resonance. Circ Arrhythm Electrophysiol 2012;5:91–100.

34. Maron BJ. Sudden death in young athletes. N Engl J Med 2003;349:1064–75.

35. Corrado D, Basso C, Schiavon M, et al. Screening for hypertrophic cardiomyopathy in young athletes. N Engl J Med 1998;339:364–9.

36. Decree of the Italian Ministry of Health, February 18, 1982. Norme per la tutela sanitaria dell'attività sportiva agonistica [rules concerning the medical protection of athletic activity]. Gazzetta Ufficiale della Repubblica Italiana. March 5, 1982:63.

37. Alcalai R, Seidman JG, Seidman CE. Genetic basis of hypertrophic cardiomyopathy: from bench to the clinics. J Cardiovasc Electrophysiol 2008;19:104–10.

38. Basso C, Thiene G, Corrado D, et al. Hypertrophic cardiomyopathy: pathologic evidence of ischemic damage in young sudden death victims. Hum Pathol 2000;31:988–98.

39. Basso C, Calabrese F, Angelini A, et al. Classification and histological, immunohistochemical, and molecular diagnosis of inflammatory myocardial disease. Heart Fail Rev 2012. [Epub ahead of print].

40. Basso C, Carturan E, Corrado D, et al. Myocarditis and dilated cardiomyopathy in athletes: diagnosis, management and recommendations for sport activity. Cardiol Clin 2007;25:423–9.

41. Thiene G, Ho SY. Aortic root pathology and sudden death in youth: review of anatomical varieties. Appl Pathol 1986;4:237–45.

42. Corrado D, Basso C, Nava A, et al. Sudden death in young people with apparently isolated mitral valve prolapse. G Ital Cardiol 1997;27:1097–105.

43. Thiene G, Pennelli N, Rossi L. Cardiac conduction system abnormalities as a possible cause of sudden death in young athletes. Hum Pathol 1983;14:704–9.

44. Basso C, Corrado D, Rossi L, et al. Ventricular preexcitation in children and young adults: atrial myocarditis as a possible trigger of sudden death. Circulation 2001;103:269–75.

45. Probst V, Kyndt F, Allouis M, et al. Genetic aspects of cardiac conduction defects. Arch Mal Coeur Vaiss 2003;96:1067–73.

46. Corrado D, Nava A, Buja G, et al. Familial cardiomyopathy underlies syndrome of right bundle branch block, ST segment elevation and sudden death. J Am Coll Cardiol 1996;27:443–8.

47. Corrado D, Basso C, Thiene G. Sudden cardiac death in young people with apparently normal heart. Cardiovasc Res 2001;50:399–408.

48. Basso C, Carturan E, Pilichou K, et al. Sudden cardiac death with normal heart: molecular autopsy. Cardiovasc Pathol 2010;19:321–5.

49. Tester DJ, Ackerman MJ. Postmortem long QT syndrome genetic testing for sudden unexplained death in the young. J Am Coll Cardiol 2007;49:240–6.

50. Crotti L, Celano G, Dagradi F, et al. Congenital long QT syndrome. Orphanet J Rare Dis 2008;3:18.

51. Gaita F, Giustetto C, Bianchi F, et al. Short QT syndrome: pharmacological treatment. J Am Coll Cardiol 2004;43:1494–9.

52. Brugada P, Brugada J. Right bundle branch block, persistent ST segment elevation and sudden cardiac death: a distinct clinical and electrocardiographic syndrome. A multicenter report. J Am Coll Cardiol 1992;20:1391–6.

53. Martini B, Nava A, Thiene G, et al. Ventricular fibrillation without apparent heart disease: description of six cases. Am Heart J 1989;118:1203–9.

54. Corrado D, Basso C, Buja G, et al. Right bundle branch block, right precordial ST-segment elevation, and sudden death in young people. Circulation 2001;103:710–7.

55. Tiso N, Stephan DA, Nava A, et al. Identification of mutations in the cardiac ryanodine receptor gene in families affected with arrhythmogenic right ventricular cardiomyopathy type 2 (ARVD2). Hum Mol Genet 2001;10:189–94.

56. Priori S, Napolitano C, Tiso N, et al. Mutations in the cardiac ryanodine receptor gene (hRyR2) underlie catecholaminergic polymorphic ventricular tachicardia. Circulation 2001;103:196–200.

57. Bauce B, Rampazzo A, Basso C, et al. Screening for ryanodine receptor type 2 mutations in families with effort-induced polymorphic ventricular arrhythmias and sudden death: early diagnosis of asymptomatic carriers. J Am Coll Cardiol 2002;40:341–9.

58. Carturan E, Tester DJ, Brost BC, et al. Postmortem genetic testing for conventional autopsy-negative sudden unexplained death: an evaluation of different DNA extraction protocols and the feasibility of mutational analysis from archival paraffin-embedded heart tissue. Am J Clin Pathol 2008;129:391–7.

59. Montisci M, El Mazloum R, Cecchetto G, et al. Anabolic androgenic steroids abuse and cardiac death in athletes: morphological and toxicological findings in four fatal cases. Forensic Sci Int 2012;217:e13–8.

60. Thiblin I, Petersson A. Pharmacoepidemiology of anabolic androgenic steroids: a review. Fundam Clin Pharmacol 2005;19:27–44.

61. Montisci M, Basso C, Thiene G. Doping e morte improvvisa. In: Ferrara SD, editor. Doping antidoping. Padova (Italy): Piccin; 2004. p. 385–413.

62. Lucena J, Blanco M, Jurado C, et al. Cocaine-related sudden death: a prospective investigation in south-west Spain. Eur Heart J 2010;31: 318–29.

Primary Prevention of Sudden Death in Young Competitive Athletes by Preparticipation Screening

Domenico Corrado, MD, PhD[a],*, Alessandro Biffi, MD[b],
Federico Migliore, MD[a], Alessandro Zorzi, MD[a],
Ilaria Rigato, MD, PhD[a], Barbara Bauce, MD, PhD[a],
Georgiane Crespi Ponta, MD[a],
Fernando Cardoso Bianchini, MD[a], Maurizio Schiavon, MD[c],
Cristina Basso, MD, PhD[d], Gaetano Thiene, MD[d]

KEYWORDS

- Athletes • Cardiomyopathy • Electrocardiogram • Preparticipation screening • Sports cardiology
- Sudden death

KEY POINTS

- Competitive sports activity is associated with an increase in the risk of sudden cardiovascular death in susceptible adolescents and young adults with clinically silent cardiovascular disorders.
- Screening including 12-lead electrocardiogram (ECG) has been demonstrated to allow identification of athletes affected by malignant heart muscle diseases at a presymptomatic stage and to lead to substantial reduction of the risk of sudden cardiovascular death during sports (*primary prevention*).
- The use of modern criteria for interpretation of the ECG in the athlete significantly improves the screening accuracy by reducing the false-positive rate (increased specificity), with the important requisite of maintaining the ability for detection of life-threatening heart diseases (preserved sensitivity).
- Screening including ECG has a more favorable cost–benefit ratio than that based on history and physical examination alone, with cost estimates per year of life saved below the threshold allowing one to consider a health intervention to be cost effective.

INTRODUCTION

The catastrophic nature of sudden cardiac death (SCD) during sports activity mandates the medical community to develop and implement effective preventive strategies.[1–7] Preparticipation screening offers the potential to identify athletes who have life-threatening cardiovascular abnormalities before onset of symptoms and to reduce the risk of sudden death (SD) during sports

Disclosures: No conflicts of interest to declare.
Sources of funding: This study was supported by Fondazione Cariparo, Padova and Rovigo, Italy; and Registry of Cardio-Cerebro-Vascular Pathology, Veneto Region, Venice, Italy.
[a] Division of Cardiology, Department of Cardiac, Thoracic and Vascular Sciences, University of Padova, Via Giustiniani 2, 35121, Padova, Italy; [b] Department of Cardiology, Center of Sport Medicine and Science, Largo Pietro Gabrielli 1, 00197 Rome, Italy; [c] Department of Social Health, Center for Sports Medicine and Physical Activity, Via dei Colli 6, 35143, Padova, Italy; [d] Cardiovascular Pathology, Department of Cardiac, Thoracic and Vascular Sciences, University of Padova, Via A. Gabelli 61, 35121, Padova, Italy
* Corresponding author. Division of Cardiology, Department of Cardiac, Thoracic and Vascular Sciences, University of Padova, Via Giustiniani 2, 35120, Padova, Italy.
E-mail address: domenico.corrado@unipd.it

Card Electrophysiol Clin 5 (2013) 13–21
http://dx.doi.org/10.1016/j.ccep.2013.01.001

(*primary prevention of SD*). A nationwide program of systematic preparticipation evaluation of competitive athletes, essentially based on 12-lead ECG, has been the practice in Italy for 25 years.[8]

In the 1960s, the World Health Organization adopted the criteria for judging public health screening measures that were set out by Wilson and Jungner.[8] According to these criteria, a population-based screening program is justifiable when (1) the condition to be detected is of public health importance, (2) there is an effective test for detecting the condition at a sufficiently early stage to permit intervention, (3) there are available effective preventive measures/treatments for the condition when it is detected at an early stage, and (4) there is evidence that early treatment, before onset of symptoms, leads to better outcomes. This article examines whether the long-running Italian program of preparticipation cardiovascular evaluation of competitive athletes fulfilled the criteria set by Wilson and Jungner so as to be considered an efficient health strategy for prevention of SD during sports activity.

Box 1
Cardiovascular causes of sudden death associated with sports
Age ≥35 years
Coronary artery disease
Age <35 years
Hypertrophic cardiomyopathy
Arrhythmogenic right ventricular cardiomyopathy/dysplasia
Congenital anomalies of coronary arteries
Myocarditis
Aortic rupture
Valvular disease
Preexcitation syndromes
Cardiac conduction diseases
Ion channel diseases
Congenital heart disease, operated or unoperated

EPIDEMIOLOGY OF SUDDEN DEATH IN ATHLETES

The incidence of SD in young competitive athletes (≤35 years of age) varies in the different athlete series reported in the literature. The SD rate has been estimated to be less than 1 in 100,000 participants per year in US high-school and college athletes.[9,10] A prospective study in Italy reported a yearly incidence of approximately 3 per 100,000 in young competitive athletes (defined as individuals aged ≤35 years who are engaged regularly in exercise training as well as participate in official athletic competitions).[6] The risk of SD in athletes increases with age and is greater in men.[1,2,6] This fact explains why the mortality rates found in the Italian investigation were significantly higher than those reported in the United States. Compared with US high-school and college participants, the Italian athletic population included older athletes (age range 12–35 years vs 12–24 years) and a significantly higher proportion of men (82% vs 65%).

Adolescent and young adults involved in sports activity have an estimated risk of SCD that is 2.8 times greater than that of their nonathletic counterparts.[6,11] In fact, sports acts as a trigger of arrhythmic cardiac arrest in athletes who are affected by predisposing cardiovascular conditions. This finding reinforces the concept that a moral and ethical obligation exists for physicians and athletic trainers to ensure that athletes are systematically screened to identify those with potentially lethal heart diseases and to protect them against the *increased* risk of SD.

As reported in **Box 1**, the causes of SD during sports activity reflect the age of the participants. Atherosclerotic coronary artery disease accounts for the vast majority of fatalities in adults (age >35 years), while cardiomyopathies and channelopathies have been consistently identified as the leading cause of cardiac arrest in younger athletes.[1–7,12–14] In the latter age group, hypertrophic cardiomyopathy (HCM) has been reported to account for more than one-third of the fatal cases in the United States[1,5,7,9] and arrhythmogenic right ventricular cardiomyopathy (ARVC) accounts for approximately one-fourth of the fatal cases in the Veneto region of Italy.[2,4,6]

ITALIAN SCREENING PROGRAM

The flow chart of the Italian protocol for preparticipation screening is shown in **Fig. 1**. Screening usually starts at the beginning of competitive athletic activity (age 12–14 years) and is repeated on a regular basis. Screening in children is not justified because the phenotypic manifestations (both ECG abnormalities and arrhythmic substrates) of most inherited heart diseases at risk of SD are age dependent and occur during adolescence and young adulthood.[4]

The screening purpose is not to detect the small number of athletes who will eventually succumb to SD but to identify the larger cohort of athletes affected by at-risk cardiovascular diseases. Most cardiovascular conditions responsible for SD in young competitive athletes are clinically silent

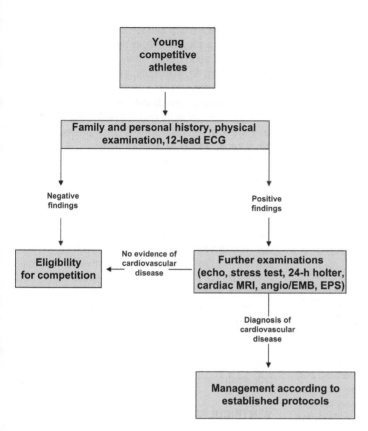

Fig. 1. Flow chart of the Italian protocol of preparticipation screening. First-line examination includes family history, physical examination, and 12-lead ECG. Additional tests are requested only for subjects who have positive findings at initial evaluation. Athletes ultimately diagnosed with cardiovascular diseases are managed according to available guidelines. Angio/EMB, contrast angiography/endomyocardial biopsy; EPS, electrophysiologic study with programed ventricular stimulation; MRI, magnetic resonance imaging. (*Modified from* Corrado D, Pelliccia A, Bjørnstad HH, et al. Cardiovascular preparticipation screening of young competitive athletes for prevention of sudden death: proposal for a common European protocol. Consensus statement of the Study Group of Sport Cardiology of the Working Group of Cardiac Rehabilitation and Exercise Physiology and the Working Group of Myocardial and Pericardial Diseases of the European Society of Cardiology. Eur Heart J 2005;26:523; with permission.)

and unlikely to be suspected or diagnosed on the basis of spontaneous symptoms.[1–7] This finding explains why a screening protocol based solely on the athlete's history and physical examination is of marginal value for identification of those with cardiac disorders at risk for SD. Preparticipation cardiovascular screening has traditionally been performed in the United States by means of history (personal and family) and physical examination, without 12-lead ECG or other testing. This screening method is currently recommended by the American Heart Association, although it has a recognized limited power to detect potentially lethal cardiovascular abnormalities in young athletes.[15] Glover and Maron found that of 134 high-school and collegiate athletes experiencing SCD who had undergone a preparticipation medical evaluation, only 3% were suspected of having cardiac disease and, eventually, less than 1% received an accurate diagnosis.[16]

Twelve-lead ECG enhances the sensitivity of the screening process by allowing early detection of cardiovascular conditions distinctively manifesting with ECG abnormalities, such as HCM, ARVC/dysplasia, dilated cardiomyopathy, Wolff-Parkinson-White syndrome, Lenègre conduction disease, long and short QT syndromes, and Brugada syndrome.[4] Overall, these conditions account for two-thirds of SDs in young competitive athletes. The Italian experience showed that ECG screening actually identifies *asymptomatic* athletes with previously undiagnosed cardiovascular abnormalities.[2–4,17,18] Among 33,735 athletes undergoing preparticipation screening at the Center for Sports Medicine in Padua, 22 (0.07%) showed definitive evidence, both clinical and echocardiographic, of HCM.[3] An absolute value of screening sensitivity for HCM cannot be derived from these data because systematic echocardiographic findings were not available. However, the 0.07% prevalence of HCM found in the white athletic population of the Veneto region of Italy, evaluated by history, physical examination, and ECG, is similar to the 0.10% prevalence reported for young white individuals in the United States, as assessed by echocardiography. This finding indicates that ECG screening may be as sensitive as echocardiographic screening in detecting HCM in the young athletic population.

Comparison between sensitivity of Italian and US screening protocols demonstrated that 12-lead ECG makes the difference. Among 22 athletes with HCM who were detected by ECG screening at the Center for Sports Medicine in Padua and disqualified from competition, only 5 (23%) would had been identified on the basis of a positive family history, symptoms, or abnormal physical findings, in the absence of an ECG.[3] Hence, the estimated sensitivity of the Italian screening modality for identification of athletes with HCM is 77% greater than that of the screening protocol (not including ECG) recommended by the American Heart Association.[4]

On the other hand, the possibility of detecting either premature coronary atherosclerosis or anomalous coronary artery in young competitive athletes is limited by the scarcity of baseline ECG signs of myocardial ischemia.[3,4]

PHYSIOLOGIC VERSUS PATHOLOGIC ABNORMALITIES IN ATHLETES' ECG

ECG changes usually develop in trained athletes as a consequence of the heart's adaptation to sustained physical exercise ("athlete's heart").[19] ECG has been traditionally considered to be a poor screening tool in the athlete, because of its presumed high level of false-positive results.[1,20,21] The Italian screening experience does not confirm this general idea that ECG is a nonspecific and non–cost-effective test. Among 42,386 athletes initially screened by history, physical examination, and 12-lead ECG, 3914 (9%) had positive findings so as to require further examination, 879 (2%) were diagnosed with cardiovascular disorders, and 91 (0.2%) were ultimately disqualified for potentially lethal heart diseases. The percentage of false-positive results, that is, athletes with a normal heart but positive screening findings, was 7% for all cardiovascular disorders and 8.8% for heart diseases at high risk of SD during sports (Fig. 2).

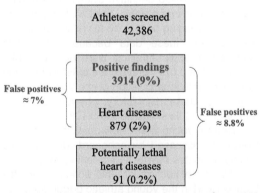

Fig. 2. Results of preparticipation screening from 1982 to 2004 at the Center for sports medicine of Padua, Italy (see the text for explanation). (*Modified from* Corrado D, Basso C, Pelliccia A, et al. Sports and heart disease. In: Camm J, Luscher TF, Serruys PW, editors. The ESC textbook of cardiovascular medicine. New York: Oxford University Press; 2009. p. 1224; with permission.)

Appropriate interpretation of ECG abnormalities has played a crucial role in the proper cardiovascular evaluation and management of Italian athletes (Fig. 3).[21] In Italy, preparticipation evaluation is performed by cardiologists and specialists in sports medicine who have specific training, medical skill, and scientific culture to reliably identify relevant familial background, clinical symptoms, and ECG abnormalities.

Recent recommendations of the European Society of Cardiology (ESC) Section of Sports Cardiology provide cardiologists and sports medicine physicians with a modern approach to distinguish between physiologic and potentially pathologic ECG patterns.[22] The ECG abnormalities are divided into 2 groups according to their prevalence, relation to exercise training, association with an increased cardiovascular risk, and need for further clinical investigation to confirm (or exclude) an underlying cardiovascular disease (see Fig. 3). Defining which ECG changes are physiologic and which are pathologic has significant favorable effects on the athlete's cardiovascular management including clinical diagnosis, risk stratification, and cost savings.[21,22]

VENTRICULAR ARRHYTHMIAS

The most common mechanism of cardiac arrest during sports activity is abrupt ventricular fibrillation (VF) or ventricular tachycardia (VT) degenerating into VF. This fact explains why demonstration of ventricular arrhythmias in the athlete's ECG is regarded as a warning sign of increased cardiovascular risk.

Ventricular arrhythmias confer adverse prognosis when underlying heart disease is present.[23–26] Systematic investigation of persons with SCD in the Veneto region of Italy demonstrated that the presence of even isolated premature ventricular beats on basal ECG at preparticipation screening may be the only clinical warning sign of heart disease at high risk of arrhythmic cardiac arrest in otherwise asymptomatic athletes.[12] The first objective of cardiovascular evaluation of an athlete with ventricular arrhythmias is to search for underlying cardiovascular disease at risk of SD.[24,26] First-line examination includes echocardiogram, 24-hour Holter monitoring, exercise testing, and signal-averaged ECG (SAECG). A careful echocardiographic evaluation of even subtle morphofunctional ventricular abnormalities is required. Twenty-four-hour Holter recordings have to be performed during periods of intense physical activity and preferably whenever the athlete is performing specific sports activity. The likelihood of underlying cardiovascular abnormalities and the arrhythmic risk increases with

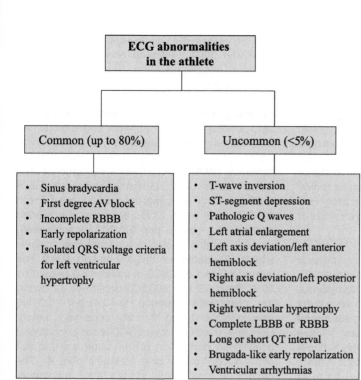

Fig. 3. Classification of ECG abnormalities in the athlete. *Common ECG abnormalities*: Up to 80% of trained athletes exhibit ECG changes such as sinus bradycardia, first-degree atrioventricular (AV) block, early repolarization, incomplete right bundle branch block (RBBB) and pure increase of QRS voltages (*Group 1*). Such common ECG changes are the consequence of the physiologic cardiovascular adaptation to sustained physical exertion and do not reflect the presence of an underlying cardiovascular disease. Therefore, they are not associated with an increase of cardiovascular risk and make an athlete eligibility for competitive sports without additional evaluation. *Uncommon ECG abnormalities*: This subset includes uncommon ECG patterns (<5%) such as ST-segment and T-wave repolarization abnormalities, pathologic Q waves, intraventricular conduction defects, and ventricular arrhythmias (*Group 2*). These ECG abnormalities are unrelated to athletic conditioning and should be regarded as an expression of possible underlying cardiovascular disorders, notably cardiomyopathies and cardiac ion channel diseases, and, thus, associated with an inherent increased risk of sudden arrhythmic death. LBBB, left bundle branch block. (*Modified from* Corrado D, Pelliccia A, Heidbuchel H, et al, on behalf of the Sections of Sports Cardiology of the European Association of Cardiovascular Prevention and Rehabilitation, Working Group of Myocardial and Pericardial Disease of the European Society of Cardiology. Recommendations for interpretation of 12-lead electrocardiogram in the athlete. Eur Heart J 2010;31:245; with permission.)

frequent and complex premature ventricular beats (>2000/24 hours), different morphologies, and couplets/nonsustained VT.[27] Exercise tests should be adapted to the specific type of exercise/sport responsible for the arrhythmic events, because a conventional exercise test may not replicate the specific clinical situation and the arrhythmogenic mechanisms produced by actively participating in the sport. Increase in the arrhythmia frequency at the beginning of exercise, disappearance at peak exercise, and reappearance during recovery usually suggest the benign nature of the ectopic ventricular rhythm. Instead, triggering or worsening of ventricular arrhythmia during exercise may point to underlying inherited cardiomyopathies or ion channel diseases and may predict malignant arrhythmic events at risk of SD during sports. A possible exception is the right ventricular outflow tract (RVOT) VT, which is characterized by repetitive monomorphic bouts of premature ventricular beats or paroxysmal sustained episodes, with the typical left bundle branch block/inferior axis pattern.[28] RVOT tachycardia is usually triggered by exercise and can be interrupted by adenosine. It is an idiopathic and

benign arrhythmic condition, provided that an underlying ARVC is carefully excluded.

The induction of polymorphic VT during exercise always carries a bad prognosis. Polymorphic VT with alternating complexes ("bidirectional" pattern), induced during exercise, suggests a specific inherited ion channel disorder, that is, "catecholaminergic polymorphic ventricular tachycardia," which predisposes to exercise-induced arrhythmic cardiac arrest in the absence of structural heart disease.[29] Registration of late potentials by the SAECG may be a sign of delayed ventricular activation and a proarrhythmogenic substrate. Positive result of SAECG has been found to be a criterion for detecting early/minor forms of ARVC and may help in the differential diagnosis of idiopathic RVOT ventricular arrhythmia.[30] There should be attempts to document a 12-lead ECG of the ventricular arrhythmias by exercise testing or 12-lead Holter monitoring. Careful assessment of the morphology of the arrhythmic QRS complex and coexistent ECG abnormalities may help to characterize the anatomic origin and the cause/mechanism of the arrhythmia. A left bundle branch morphology and inferior QRS axis (with negative QRS complexes in V1 and electrical transition between V2 and V3 or V3 and V4) is a hallmark of idiopathic RVOT ventricular arrhythmias. Similar morphology but with earlier precordial transition may indicate origin in the left ventricular (LV) outflow tract.

A rare clinical entity is ventricular arrhythmia with a borderline width QRS ($\leq$0.12 seconds) and a right bundle branch block/superior axis pattern, which is pathognomonic for origin in the left posterior fascicle (the so-called fascicular ventricular tachycardia).[31] This entity carries no adverse prognosis unless associated with syncope during exercise or heart disease.

The analysis of concomitant repolarization/depolarization ECG abnormalities may provide relevant information to interpret the clinical significance of a documented ventricular arrhythmia. The association between a premature ventricular beat with a left bundle branch block pattern and repolarization abnormalities, such as T-wave inversion in right precordial leads is highly suggestive of ARVC.[22] The coexistence of a right ventricular (RV) conduction defect in the form of a prolonged QRS duration or a delayed S-wave upstroke in V1 to V3 further increases the likelihood of an ARVC.[32] On the other hand, premature ventricular beats originating from the LV, associated with negative T waves in the left precordial leads, must raise the suspicion of an LV heart muscle disease such as dilated/inflammatory cardiomyopathy, HCM, LV noncompaction, or a predominantly left-sided ARVC.

In selected athletes in whom previous clinical and instrumental findings are inconclusive, contrast-enhanced cardiovascular magnetic resonance imaging, nuclear scintigraphy, or other invasive tests such as electrophysiological study, ventriculocoronary angiography, and endomyocardial biopsy may be required to achieve a definite diagnosis. Molecular genetic studies are increasingly available for preclinical diagnosis of inherited arrhythmogenic heart muscle diseases, including channelopathies.[4,22–24]

Workup should also include a search for agents that may enhance electrical ventricular irritability, such as the use of excessive amount of alcohol, illicit drugs, or stimulants, particularly ephedrine and caffeine.

SCREENING EFFICACY FOR PREVENTION OF SUDDEN DEATH

The long-term Italian experience has provided compelling evidence that ECG screening is a lifesaving strategy. A time–trend analysis of the incidence of SCD in young competitive athletes aged 12 to 35 years in the Veneto region of Italy between 1979 and 2004 confirmed and extended these previous observations on athletes' outcome.[18] The long-term impact of the Italian screening program on prevention of SCD in athletes was assessed by comparing temporal trends in SCD among screened athletes and unscreened nonathletes. Assessed intervals were prescreening (1979–1981), early screening (1982–1992), and late screening (1993–2004). The analysis demonstrated a sharp decline of SCD in athletes after the introduction of the nationwide screening program in 1982. A total of 55 SCDs occurred in screened athletes (1.9 deaths per 100,000 person-years), and 265 deaths occurred in unscreened nonathletes (0.79 deaths per 100,000 person-years). The annual incidence of SCD in athletes decreased by 89%, from 3.6 per 100,000 person-years during the prescreening period to 0.4 per 100,000 person-years during the late screening period. However, the incidence of SCD in the unscreened nonathletic population of the same age did not change significantly over that time (**Fig. 4**). The decline in death rate started after mandatory screening was launched and persisted to the late screening period. Compared with the prescreening period (1979–1981), the relative risk of SCD was 44% lower in the early screening period (1982–1992) and 79% lower in the late screening period (1993–2004). It is noteworthy that most of the reduced death rate was due to fewer cases of SD from cardiomyopathies. Most of the reduction was attributable to fewer deaths from HCM and ARVC. A parallel analysis of the causes of disqualifications from competitive sports at the Center for Sports Medicine in the Padua country area showed that the proportion of athletes identified and disqualified for cardiomyopathies doubled from the early to the late screening period. This finding indicates that mortality reduction was a reflection of a lower incidence of SD from cardiomyopathies, as a result of increasing identification over time of affected athletes at preparticipation screening.

TREATMENT OF ATHLETES DIAGNOSED WITH HEART DISEASES AT AN EARLY STAGE

The importance of identification of asymptomatic athletes with cardiovascular diseases by ECG screening relies on the concrete possibility of SD prevention by lifestyle modification, including restriction of competitive sports activity, and concomitant prophylactic treatment with antiarrhythmic drugs, β-blockers, and implantable cardioverter-defibrillator therapy. Athletes disqualified for cardiovascular reasons have a good prognosis over a long-term follow-up.[3,18] In this

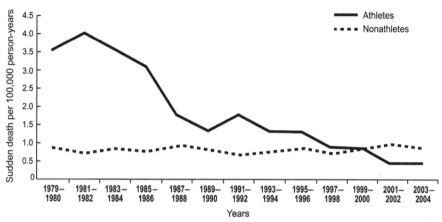

Fig. 4. Annual incidence rates of SCD per 100,000 person-years, among screened competitive athletes and unscreened nonathletes aged 12 to 35 years in the Veneto region of Italy, from 1979 to 2004. During the study period (the nationwide preparticipation screening program was launched in 1982), the annual incidence of SCD declined by 89% in screened athletes (*P* for trend <.001). In contrast, the incidence rate of SCD did not demonstrate consistent changes over time in unscreened nonathletes. (*Modified from* Corrado D, Basso C, Pavei A, et al. Trends in sudden cardiovascular death in young competitive athletes after implementation of a preparticipation screening program. JAMA 2006;296:1596; with permission.)

regard, none of the 22 asymptomatic athletes who were disqualified for HCM died during an average 7.8-year follow-up period. Of note, 3 of these former athletes with HCM later experienced serious arrhythmic complications that were successfully treated by β-blockers and/or amiodarone. Thus, these athletes actually carried an increased arrhythmic risk and their favorable long-term outcome was the result of both restriction from competitive sports and the subsequent close follow-up and clinical management.

SCREENING COST AND FEASIBILITY

The long-term Italian experience indicates that screening is feasible because of its limited costs in the setting of a mass program.[3,32] The cost of performing a preparticipation cardiac history/physical examination by qualified physicians has been estimated to be ≈20 Euro per athlete and increases to ≈30 Euro per athlete if a 12-lead ECG is added. The screening cost is covered by the athlete or by the athletic team, except for athletes younger than 18 years, for whom the expense is supported by the National Health System.

The cost of further evaluation of athletes with positive findings at first-line examination is lesser than expected because of the *presumed* low specificity of their ECG. The long-running Italian screening program showed that the percentage of false-positive results (ie, athletes with a normal heart but positive screening findings) requiring additional testing, mainly echocardiography, did

not exceed 9%, with a modest proportional impact on cost (see **Fig. 2**).[18]

The demographics of the screened athletic population, consisting of adolescents and young adults, as well as the genetic nature of the leading causes of SD in this age group, profoundly affects cost–benefit considerations.[33] Unlike older patients with coronary artery diseases or heart failure, young individuals diagnosed with a genetic disease at risk of arrhythmic cardiac arrest will survive for many decades with normal or nearly normal life expectancy, thanks to restriction from competition and prophylactic therapy against life-threatening arrhythmias.[3] This large amount of life-years saved favorably influences cost-effectiveness analysis of the screening process.

Furthermore, the identification by preparticipation screening of index athletes with inherited heart diseases enables cascade screening of relatives, which may lead to identification of other affected family members and save additional lives.[33,34]

CONCLUSIONS AND FUTURE DIRECTIONS

According to the long-term Italian experience, preparticipation cardiovascular evaluation of competitive athletes is a lifesaving strategy that meets the following criteria set by Wilson and Jungner[8] for appraising the validity of a screening program: (1) safe sports activity represents an important health issue; (2) affected, but still asymptomatic, athletes are accurately identified by ECG screening; (3) an effective management strategy exists based on restriction of life-threatening training/competition and subsequent clinical treatment; and (4) most importantly, early identification and management of asymptomatic athletes favorably modify the outcome of the underlying diseases leading to substantial reduction of SD.

In future, prospective epidemiologic studies in countries other than Italy are warranted to evaluate specific SCD rate, to explore whether genetic and/or environmental factors may influence the prevalence and the nature of cardiovascular causes of sport-related death, and to assess the costs and the accuracy of screening testing as well as the efficacy of recommendations to limit sports participation. The use of updated ECG criteria is expected to improve ECG accuracy in the evaluation of trained athletes, leading to a lower proportion of false-positive results and considerable cost savings in the context of a preparticipation screening process. Further studies are needed to test the accuracy of ECG screening, in relation to gender, age, ethnicity, and different level of training and/or type of sports. Specifically, the utility and cost-effectiveness of exercise test for screening middle-aged and senior athletes engaged in leisure-time sports activity remains to be demonstrated.

REFERENCES

1. Maron BJ. Sudden death in young athletes. N Engl J Med 2003;349:1064–75.
2. Corrado D, Basso C, Thiene G. Essay: sudden death in young athletes. Lancet 2005;366:S47–8.
3. Corrado D, Basso C, Schiavon M, et al. Screening for hypertrophic cardiomyopathy in young athletes. N Engl J Med 1998;339:364–9.
4. Corrado D, Pelliccia A, Bjørnstad HH, et al. Cardiovascular preparticipation screening of young competitive athletes for prevention of sudden death: proposal for a common European protocol. Consensus statement of the Study Group of Sport Cardiology of the Working Group of Cardiac Rehabilitation and Exercise Physiology and the Working Group of Myocardial and Pericardial Diseases of the European Society of Cardiology. Eur Heart J 2005;26: 516–24.
5. Van Camp SP, Bloor CM, Mueller FO, et al. Nontraumatic sports death in high school and college athletes. Med Sci Sports Exerc 1995;27:641–7.
6. Corrado D, Basso C, Rizzoli G, et al. Does sports activity enhance the risk of sudden death in adolescents and young adults? J Am Coll Cardiol 2003;42: 1959–63.
7. Burke AP, Farb A, Virmani R, et al. Sports-related and non-sports-related sudden cardiac death in young adults. Am Heart J 1991;121:568–75.
8. Wilson JM, Jungner G. Principles and practice of screening for diseases. Geneva (Switzerland): WHO Publication; 1968.
9. Maron BJ, Doerer JJ, Haas TS, et al. Sudden deaths in young competitive athletes: analysis of 1866 deaths in the United States, 1980-2006. Circulation 2009;119:1085–92.
10. Maron BJ, Haas TS, Doerer JJ, et al. Comparison of U.S. and Italian experiences with sudden cardiac deaths in young competitive athletes and implications for preparticipation screening strategies. Am J Cardiol 2009;15(104):276–80.
11. Corrado D, Migliore F, Basso C, et al. Exercise and the risk of sudden cardiac death. Herz 2006;31: 553–8.
12. Corrado D, Thiene G, Nava A, et al. Sudden death in young competitive athletes: clinicopathologic correlations in 22 cases. Am J Med 1990;89:588–96.
13. Corrado D, Migliore F, Zorzi A, et al. Sudden cardiac death and preparticipation sports screening. In: Elzouki AY, Harfi HA, Nazer HM, et al, editors. Textbook of clinical pediatrics. Berlin, Heidelberg (Germany): Springer; 2012. p. 2399–412.
14. Corrado D, Pelliccia A, Antzelevitch C, et al. ST segment elevation and sudden death in the athlete. In: Antzelevitch C, editor. The Brugada syndrome: from bench to bedside. Oxford (United Kingdom): Blackwell Futura; 2005. p. 119–29.
15. Maron BJ, Thompson PD, Ackerman MJ, et al. Recommendations and considerations related to preparticipation screening for cardiovascular abnormalities in competitive athletes: 2007 update. A scientific statement from the American Heart Association Council on Nutrition, Physical Activity, and Metabolism: endorsed by the American College of Cardiology Foundation. Circulation 2007;115: 1643–55.
16. Glower DW, Maron BJ. Profile of preparticipation cardiovascular screening for high school athletes. JAMA 1998;279:1817–9.
17. Pelliccia A, Di Paolo FM, Corrado D, et al. Evidence for efficacy of the Italian national pre-participation screening programme for identification of hypertrophic cardiomyopathy in competitive athletes. Eur Heart J 2006;27:2196–200.
18. Corrado D, Basso C, Pavei A, et al. Trends in sudden cardiovascular death in young competitive athletes after implementation of a preparticipation screening program. JAMA 2006;296:1593–601.
19. Maron BJ, Pelliccia A. The heart of trained athletes: cardiac remodeling and the risks of sports, including sudden death. Circulation 2006;114: 1633–44.
20. Pelliccia A, Maron BJ, Culasso F, et al. Clinical significance of abnormal electrocardiographic patterns in trained athletes. Circulation 2000;102:278–84.

21. Corrado D, McKenna WJ. Appropriate interpretation of the athlete's electrocardiogram saves lives as well as money. Eur Heart J 2007;28:1920–2.

22. Corrado D, Pelliccia A, Heidbuchel H, et al, on behalf of the Sections of Sports Cardiology of the European Association of Cardiovascular Prevention and Rehabilitation, Working Group of Myocardial and Pericardial Disease of the European Society of Cardiology. Recommendations for interpretation of 12-lead electrocardiogram in the athlete. Eur Heart J 2010;31:243–59.

23. Corrado D, Basso C, Pelliccia A, et al. Sports and heart disease. In: Camm J, Luscher TF, Serruys PW, editors. The ESC textbook of cardiovascular medicine. New York: Oxford University Press; 2009. p. 1215–37.

24. Pelliccia A, Fagard R, Bjornstad HH, et al. Recommendations for competitive sports participation in athletes with cardiovascular disease: a consensus document from the Study Group of Sports Cardiology of the Working Group of Cardiac Rehabilitation and Exercise Physiology and the Working Group of Myocardial and Pericardial Diseases of the European Society of Cardiology. Eur Heart J 2005;26:1422–45.

25. Maron BJ, Zipes DP. 36th Bethesda Conference: recommendations for determining eligibility for competition in athletes with cardiovascular abnormalities. J Am Coll Cardiol 2005;45:1373–5.

26. Heidbüchel H, Corrado D, Biffi A, et al, Study Group on Sports Cardiology of the European Association for Cardiovascular Prevention and Rehabilitation. Recommendations for participation in leisure-time physical activity and competitive sports of patients with arrhythmias and potentially arrhythmogenic conditions. Part II: ventricular arrhythmias, channelopathies and implantable defibrillators. Eur J Cardiovasc Prev Rehabil 2006;13:676–86.

27. Biffi A, Pelliccia A, Verdile L, et al. Long-term clinical significance of frequent and complex ventricular tachyarrhythmias in trained athletes. J Am Coll Cardiol 2002;40:446–52.

28. Lerman BB, Stein K, Engelstein ED, et al. Mechanism of repetitive monomorphic ventricular tachycardia. Circulation 1995;92:421–9.

29. Bauce B, Rampazzo A, Basso C, et al. Screening for ryanodine receptor type 2 mutations in families with effort-induced polymorphic ventricular arrhythmias and sudden death: early diagnosis of asymptomatic carriers. J Am Coll Cardiol 2002;40:341–9.

30. Corrado D, Basso C, Leoni L, et al. Three-dimensional electroanatomical voltage mapping and histologic evaluation of myocardial substrate in right ventricular outflow tract tachycardia. J Am Coll Cardiol 2008;51:731–9.

31. Lin D, Hsia HH, Gerstenfeld EP, et al. Idiopathic fascicular left ventricular tachycardia: linear ablation lesion strategy for noninducible or nonsustained tachycardia. Heart Rhythm 2005;2:934–9.

32. Turrini P, Corrado D, Basso C, et al. Dispersion of ventricular depolarization-repolarization: a noninvasive marker for risk stratification in arrhythmogenic right ventricular cardiomyopathy. Circulation 2001;103:3075–80.

33. Myerburg RJ, Vetter VL. Electrocardiograms should be included in preparticipation screening of athletes. Circulation 2007;116:2616–26.

34. Corrado D, Basso C, Schiavon M, et al. Pre-participation screening of young competitive athletes for prevention of sudden cardiac death. J Am Coll Cardiol 2008;52:1981–9.

Secondary Prevention of Sudden Death in Athletes
The Essential Role of Automated External Defibrillators

Ashwin L. Rao, MD[a],*, Irfan M. Asif, MD[b],
Jonathan A. Drezner, MD[c]

KEYWORDS

- Sudden cardiac death • Cardiac arrest • Public access defibrillation • Emergency planning

KEY POINTS

- Sudden cardiac arrest (SCA) is the leading cause of death in exercising young athletes.
- Automated external defibrillators (AEDs) are an integral link in the "chain of survival" and their prompt use promotes higher survival rates from SCA.
- Public access defibrillation (PAD) programs shorten the time interval between SCA and shock delivery and train likely responders in cardiopulmonary resuscitation (CPR) and AED use.
- SCA should be assumed in any collapsed and unresponsive athlete.
- Prompt management of SCA, including rapid recognition of SCA, immediate initiation of chest compressions, and retrieval and use of an AED as soon as possible can be life saving for athletes with SCA.

INTRODUCTION

The sudden loss of life from cardiac arrest is a tragic event with broad reach and impact. More than 300,000 individuals die annually from sudden cardiac arrest (SCA) in the United States, and historically, the rate of survival from these events is poor.[1–5] In recent years, media coverage has focused attention on athletic cardiac arrest, in cases of both death (ie, Miklos Feher, Wes Leonard, and Hank Gathers) and survival (ie, Fabrice Muamba, Anthony Van Loo, and Jiri Fischer). Cases of SCA in athletes typically raise questions regarding proper emergency planning for such events and the role of automated external defibrillators (AEDs) at sporting venues.

The strongest determinant of survival from SCA is the time from arrest to defibrillation. Survival drops by 7% to 10% with each minute that defibrillation is delayed.[6] Several studies evaluating public access defibrillation (PAD) programs in areas of high population density have demonstrated improved survival rates from SCA.[7–10] PAD programs shorten the time between cardiac arrest and shock delivery to restore spontaneous circulation. Publicly available AEDs have been particularly helpful in areas where the emergency medical service (EMS) call-to-shock interval cannot be consistently achieved within 5 minutes of SCA.[8,9,11] This article reviews strategies for effective secondary prevention of sudden death in athletes and the critical role of AEDs.

Disclosures: No conflicts of interest to declare.
[a] Department of Family Medicine, Hall Health Primary Care Center, University of Washington, Box 354410, 4060 East Stevens Way, Seattle, WA 98195, USA; [b] Department of Family Medicine, The University of Tennessee, 1924 Alcoa Highway, Knoxville, TN 37920-6999, USA; [c] Department of Family Medicine, University of Washington, Box 354410, 4060 East Stevens Way, Seattle, WA 98195, USA
* Corresponding author.
E-mail address: ashwin@fammed.washington.edu

Card Electrophysiol Clin 5 (2013) 23–31
http://dx.doi.org/10.1016/j.ccep.2012.11.004

SUDDEN DEATH IN ATHLETES: WHAT IS THE RISK?

SCA is the leading cause of death in exercising young athletes.[12] In the United States, a minimum estimate of between 100 and 150 cases of SCA occur per year in competitive athletes.[13] Studies consistently show that 0.2% to 0.7% of competitive athletes harbor underlying cardiovascular disease associated with SCA.[14–21] Causes of sudden cardiac death (SCD) in athletes include diseases that affect the myocardium, coronary arteries, and proximal aorta, and primary electrical diseases (Table 1). Intense physical exercise places mechanical and metabolic stresses on the cardiovascular system and can produce lethal ventricular arrhythmias in athletes with pathologic cardiac disease. Studies demonstrated that competitive young athletes are 2.8 to 4.5 times more likely to die from SCA than age-matched peers, and more than 80% of SCD in athletes occurs in relation to physical exertion.[12,14,22]

Corrado and colleagues[23] reported the incidence of SCD in athletes aged 12 to 35 to be 3.6/100,000 athletes per year before implementation of a nationwide screening program. Within the United States, the exact incidence of SCA in young athletes is unknown. Initial estimates of SCD of 0.3 to 0.6 per 100,000 athletes per year relied heavily on media reports, catastrophic insurance claims, and other nonmandatory databases to identify cases and likely underestimate the true magnitude of the problem.[12,24,25] Defining the incidence of SCA/SCD in any population requires both the capacity to accurately identify cases and a defined study population. In recent years, several studies have used more rigorous methodology reliant on these principles to estimate the incidence of SCA in selected active populations (Table 2).[12,21,23–32] Using a mandatory reporting system and autopsy-based study from the Department of Defense, Eckart and colleagues[26] reported an incidence of SCD in US military personnel aged 18 to 35 of 1/25,000 persons per year. Atkins and colleagues[27] studied all cases of out-of-hospital cardiac arrest with EMS response in 11 North American cities demonstrating an SCA incidence of 3.75/100,000 for individuals aged 14 to 24. Meyer and colleagues[28] recently conducted a 30-year review of SCA in individuals younger than 35 years of age from King County, Washington, using an EMS Cardiac Arrest Database. The incidence of SCA in adolescents and young adults aged 14 to 24 was 1.44/100,000.

In US competitive athletes, the rate of SCA may be higher than in studies of the general population. Drezner and colleagues[33] reported an annual SCA incidence of 4.4/100,000 in competitive high school athletes based on a cross-sectional survey of 1710 high schools. Harmon and colleagues[29] reported on the incidence of sudden death in National Collegiate Athletic Association (NCAA) athletes between 2004 and 2008. In that 5-year period, SCD was the leading medical cause of death in collegiate athletes, accounting for 76% of cases of SCD during exertion and 16% of all-cause mortality. The annual incidence of SCD in all athletes was 2.28/100,000 athletes per year, with higher rates in males (3.0/100,000) and black athletes (5.89/100,000). Notably, the rate of

Table 1 Causes of sudden cardiac death in athletes	
	Specific Cardiac Pathology
Myocardium	Hypertrophic cardiomyopathy (HCM) Arrhythmogenic right ventricular cardiomyopathy (ARVC) Dilated cardiomyopathy (DCM) Myocarditis
Coronary arteries	Anomalous origin coronary arteries Premature atherosclerosis
Primary electrical diseases	Long QT syndrome Short QT syndrome Catecholaminergic polymorphic ventricular tachycardia (CPVT) Brugada syndrome Wolff-Parkinson-White syndrome (WPW)
Proximal aorta	Marfan syndrome – aortic rupture Aortopathy associated with bicuspid aortic valve Aortic stenosis
Traumatic	Commotio cordis

Table 2
Incidence of sudden cardiac death

Population	Age	Methods and Reporting System	Incidence
US athletes			
Van Camp et al,[25] 1995	13–24	Media reports	1:300,000
Maron et al,[24] 1998	13–19	Insurance claims	1:200,000
Drezner et al,[69] 2005	18–23	Retrospective survey	1:67,000
Maron et al,[12] 2009	12–35	Media Reports, electronic databases	1:166,000
Drezner & Corrado,[21] 2011	14–17	Cross-sectional survey	1:23,000
Harmon et al,[29] 2011	17–24	NCAA Resolutions list, media reports	1:44,000
US military			
Eckart et al,[31] 2004	18–35	Mandatory	1:9000
Eckart et al,[26] 2011	18–35	Mandatory, Department of Defense	1:25,000
US adolescents			
Chugh et al,[78] 2009	10–14	Prospective, EMS/Hospital database	1:58,000
Meyer et al,[28] 2012	14–24	Prospective, EMS database	1:69,000
Italian athletes			
Corrado et al,[23] 2006	12–35	Mandatory registry	1:25,000
Norwegian athletes			
Solberg et al,[30] 2010	15–34	Mandatory, forensic registry	1:111,000
Israeli athletes			
Steinvil et al,[32] 2011	12–44	Newspaper reports	1:38,000

Abbreviations: EMS, emergency medical services; NCAA, National Collegiate Athletic Association.

SCD was alarmingly high in basketball athletes (14.3/100,000) regardless of ethnicity.

LIMITATIONS OF PRIMARY PREVENTION STRATEGIES

Customary practice for preparticipation screening within the United States uses a comprehensive personal and family history and physical examination. The American Heart Association (AHA) supports cardiovascular screening as "justifiable, necessary, and compelling on the basis of ethical, legal, and medical grounds," while also acknowledging that screening by history and physical examination may be encumbered by a high number of false-negative results.[20] Lack of physician infrastructure to properly evaluate electrocardiograms (ECGs) and the downstream costs of false-positive results are frequently cited barriers to widespread implementation of ECGs as a standard component of screening within the United States.[34,35]

In contrast, the European Society for Cardiology, International Olympic Committee, and Federation de Internationale Football Association (FIFA) recommend including the ECG as part of the standard preparticipation evaluation.[36–38] ECG greatly increases the sensitivity to detect cardiac disorders associated with SCD. The combined sensitivity from 4 recent studies to identify athletes with at-risk conditions using history and physical alone was 12% compared with 88% when using ECG.[13,15,18,19,39–41]

Initiatives are under way to train physicians on ECG interpretation to better distinguish physiologic adaptations in athletes from findings suggestive of an underlying pathologic cardiac condition.[42–44] Drezner and colleagues[44] demonstrated that physicians with little experience in ECG interpretation in athletes can greatly improve their ability to accurate classify an ECG as normal or abnormal with use of a standardized criteria tool.

No screening protocol will detect all cases of underlying cardiovascular pathology. Specifically, ECG screening will fail to identify coronary artery disease, coronary artery anomalies, and aortic root disorders, and screening does not protect against new cases of myocarditis or commotio cordis.[45] Given the limits of primary prevention and that SCA is the first manifestation of cardiac disease in 60% to 80% of young athletes with sudden death,[41] effective strategies for management of SCA are critical.

AEDS AND SECONDARY PREVENTION OF SUDDEN DEATH

Historically, survival following out-of-hospital SCA is less than 8%.[2–6] The most common initial rhythm in SCA is ventricular fibrillation (VF), in which early defibrillation is linked to improved survival.[46–49] The goal of defibrillation is to terminate ventricular fibrillation and restore spontaneous circulation. Prompt cardiopulmonary resuscitation (CPR) improves survival by lengthening the time frame in which defibrillation may be effective.[50–52] The probability of successful defibrillation diminishes rapidly over time, as VF tends to deteriorate to asystole.[53–55]

AEDs offer a simple, portable, and effective way to provide a defibrillating shock to victims of SCA and have been included in resuscitation guidelines since 2000.[11] Advances in technology have made AEDs less costly, smaller, and easier to use. Through increased availability, AEDs have allowed lay and trained rescuers to provide defibrillation at athletic venues before the arrival of EMS. AEDs are safe and accurate in identifying life-threatening ventricular tachyarrhythmias from other more benign cardiac rhythms.[56]

PAD programs place publicly available AEDs in targeted areas with a high incidence of SCA. PAD programs allow individuals other than trained public safety personnel to respond rapidly to SCA. Studies performed in a wide range of settings have demonstrated that PAD programs are effective in sites of high population density where EMS response may be slow. A recent 10-year PAD program in Los Angeles, California, found that 66% of cardiac arrests had shockable rhythms and 77% of these patients achieved return of spontaneous circulation through early defibrillation, and 69% survived to hospital discharge.[10] Other studies of PAD programs also demonstrate high survival rates in casinos (48%), airlines (36%), and airports (52%).[7–10]

AED programs have been increasingly used in the athletic setting. An early study by Drezner and Rogers[57] evaluated survival following SCA in 9 NCAA collegiate athletes. The study identified only one survivor and characterized important challenges to the prompt recognition of SCA in athletes. Drezner and colleagues[33] subsequently reported the outcomes of SCA in a cross-sectional study of 1710 US high schools with onsite AED programs. The study identified 36 cases of SCA, 14 in high school student athletes with a mean age of 16 years. An AED was deployed in 30 of 36 cases, with a 64% survival documented in both student-athletes and older nonstudents. More recently, Drezner and colleagues[58] have reported the

outcomes of SCA from a 2-year prospective study of 2149 high schools; 87% of participating schools had an onsite AED program. During the study period, 59 cases of SCA were reported, including 26 cases in students and 33 cases in adults. A defibrillator was applied in 85% of cases and a shock was delivered in 66%. Overall, 71% of SCA victims survived to hospital discharge. Notably, 89% of students and adults who developed SCA during sports or physical activity survived to hospital discharge. These studies highlight the effectiveness of early defibrillation and the importance of having onsite AEDs in the athletic setting.

EMERGENCY PLANNING FOR SCA

The ability to respond to SCA relies heavily on preparation and a coordinated effort of the responders. In 2002, the National Athletic Trainers Association (NATA) released a position statement recommending that any institution sponsoring athletic activities should develop and implement a written emergency action plan for SCA, including the acquisition of necessary equipment and training personnel in CPR and AED use.[59] In 2004, the AHA issued a consensus statement recommending that any school that could not reliably achieve an EMS call-to-shock interval of less than 5 minutes should have an onsite AED program, and in 2007 an Inter-Association Task Force provided consensus recommendations for the management of SCA in college and high school athletic programs.[60–62]

Elements for an effective AED program include (1) development of an effective communication system to alert onsite responders and activate the local EMS system; (2) coordination of the response plan among school, team, or club staff and local EMS; (3) instruction and training of potential first responders in CPR and AED use; (4) rapid availability of AEDs; and (5) practice and review of the emergency response plan at least annually. Steps also should be taken to ensure appropriate device maintenance and readiness checks before sporting events.

RECOGNITION AND MANAGEMENT OF SCA

The AHA has defined a "chain of survival" in the management of SCA[11]:

- Early recognition of SCA and activation of EMS
- Early implementation of CPR
- Early AED placement and delivery of a shock
- Early advanced life support

The approach to a collapsed and unresponsive individual in the field has traditionally involved an "Airway-Breathing-Circulation" (A-B-C) assessment by a responder trained in basic life support (BLS). The 2005 and recently revised 2010 BLS guidelines have de-emphasized the traditional "look, listen, and feel" approach stressed in prior guidelines in favor of identifying unresponsiveness in a collapsed victim.[63,64] Agonal or gasping respirations may be a sign of SCA and should not prevent initiation of CPR. Moreover, lay rescuer assessment of pulse has been eliminated because of frequent misinterpretation. Seizurelike activity may be observed in as many as 50% of athletes with SCA.[33] Thus, any myoclonic movements in a collapsed and unresponsive athlete must be assumed to signal SCA and not be mistaken for a seizure.

Steps in the "chain of survival" must be taken rapidly to improve survival from SCA. When 2 or more rescuers are present, activation of EMS, initiation of CPR, and retrieval of the AED can occur simultaneously.

In 2010, an International Consensus on Cardiopulmonary Resuscitation and Emergency Cardiovascular Care revised the recommended sequence of resuscitation from A-B-C to C-A-B (Chest compressions-Airway-Breathing).[63,64] BLS protocols now stress that all rescuers, trained or novice, should begin with chest compressions, emphasizing a circulation-first model. High-quality chest compressions involve a depth of 2 inches at a rate of 100 compressions per minute, and allow for full chest recoil. Hands-only CPR without rescue breathing is recommended for lay rescuers to simplify the rescue effort. Trained medical responders are advised to begin with chest compressions followed by ventilation, using a compression-to-ventilation ratio of 30:2.

Interruptions in chest compression should be minimized. Current research supports a 1-shock sequence (rather than 3 stacked shocks) with immediate provision of chest compressions after shock delivery without delays for rhythm reanalysis.[65,66] This promotes coronary perfusion to an otherwise stunned myocardium after defibrillation and decreases the reoccurrence of VF. CPR should be completed for 5 cycles (approximately 2 minutes) before reanalyzing the cardiac rhythm. If a nonshockable rhythm is detected, CPR should be resumed until advanced life support can be provided.

RESPONDING TO SCA IN ATHLETIC VENUES: MORE THAN JUST THE ATHLETE

Sporting arenas typically gather other individuals at risk for SCA. Emergency planning and AEDs at sporting venues offer the potential for effective secondary prevention of SCD not only for athletes, but also for spectators, coaches, referees, and other persons present at the arena. SCA can be triggered during periods of intense emotion during sports matches.[67,68] In collegiate athletic venues, up to 77% of reported SCA cases occurred in older nonathletes.[69] The frequency of SCA in adult spectators at large sporting arenas is approximately 1 in 600,000 per event, suggesting that emergency preparations should extend beyond the athlete participants and may take additional planning.[70]

BARRIERS
Cost

Despite the mounting evidence of the impact of AED programs on survival from SCA in the athletic setting, multiple obstacles remain to their successful implementation at the amateur and professional levels. Cost remains a principal factor to implementation of AEDs in youth sporting venues and schools. School budget allocations present challenging decisions on how to distribute strained resources when considering programs compared with other school initiatives. A 2007 study by Rothmier and colleagues[71] suggested that nearly 60% of AEDs in Washington State high schools were funded through donation rather than by school resources. Organizations that consider implementing AED programs must factor in the cost of the AED device itself, annual maintenance, replacement parts, and CPR and AED training for anticipated responders.[60]

Implementation

Having an AED in place is not enough to successfully prepare for an SCA event. AEDs must be implemented as part of a comprehensive emergency response plan for SCA. Data suggest that only 75% of coaches at the high school level are trained in CPR, and only 46% of schools with an AED program practice and review their plan annually.[21] The prevalence of AEDs at collegiate athletic venues (81%–91%) and European professional sporting arenas (72%) further highlight the inadequacies of cardiovascular emergency preparedness.[69,70]

Greater staff awareness of AEDs, education on recognition of SCA, and broader personnel training in CPR and AED are needed within the athletic setting to further improve outcomes from SCA. FIFA recently took the unprecedented step to require that every FIFA-sponsored football pitch be equipped with an AED.[72] The National Football

League Players Association recently provided support for education and implementation of AED programs at American football playing fields at all levels of competition. Despite compelling evidence to support the availability of onsite AED programs, only 16 of 50 states in the United States require the placement of AEDs in schools.[73]

Improving Rescuer Knowledge on AEDs

Lay rescuers can successfully use AEDs in emergency situations without harm or injury to patients, bystanders, or themselves.[74] Unfortunately, there are still many obstacles to efficient PAD programs. Schober and colleagues[75] found that more than half of 1018 lay responders could not properly identify an AED and only 47% stated they would use an AED during a cardiac arrest. There is need for increased public knowledge regarding the use, safety, and placement of AEDs. Recent investigations, including the development of mobile applications with AED "maps," have sought to identify novel methods for lay rescuers to locate nearby AEDs in case of an emergency.[76] Modern telemedical advancements (ie, smart phones and wireless Internet devices), offer the potential to strengthen links in the chain of survival.[77] In the athletic setting, AED placement and knowledge of AED location should be strongly emphasized for anticipated first responders to a cardiac emergency.

SUMMARY

SCD in young athletes is a catastrophic event that largely can be avoided through comprehensive emergency planning and preparation. The athletic community is uniquely positioned to have trained rescuers and AEDs available to respond rapidly to SCA. Proper emergency planning and implementation of new resuscitation guidelines will improve survival from SCA in the athletic setting. SCA should be suspected in any athlete who has collapsed and is unresponsive. Early recognition of SCA, prompt initiation of chest compressions, and rapid deployment of an AED are critical for the successful prevention of sudden death in athletes.

REFERENCES

1. Hazinski MF, Idris AH, Kerber RE, et al, American Heart Association Emergency Cardiovascular Committee; Council on Cardiopulmonary, Perioperative, and Critical Care; Council on Clinical Cardiology. Lay rescuer automated external defibrillator ("public access defibrillation") programs: lessons learned from an international multicenter trial: advisory statement from the American Heart Association Emergency Cardiovascular Committee; the Council on Cardiopulmonary, Perioperative, and Critical Care; and the Council on Clinical Cardiology. Circulation 2005;111(24):3336–40.
2. Becker LB, Ostrander MP, Barrett J, et al. Outcome of CPR in a large metropolitan area: where are the survivors. Ann Emerg Med 1991;20:355–61.
3. Lombardi G, Gallagher J, Gennis P. Outcome of out of hospital cardiac arrest in NYC: a pre-hospital arrest study. JAMA 1994;271:678–83.
4. Nichol G, Thomas E, Callaway CW, et al, Resuscitation Outcomes Consortium Investigators. Regional variation in out-of-hospital cardiac arrest incidence and outcome. JAMA 2008;300:1423–31.
5. Sasson C, Rogers MA, Dahl J, et al. Predictors of survival from out-of-hospital cardiac arrest: a systematic review and meta-analysis. Circ Cardiovasc Qual Outcomes 2009;3:63–8.
6. Cummins RO, Ornato JP, Thics WH, et al. Improving survival from sudden cardiac arrest: the "chain of survival" concept: a statement for health care professionals from the Advanced Cardiac Care Committee, American Heart Association. Circulation 1991;83:832–47.
7. Page RL, Joglar JA, Kowal RC, et al. Use of automated external defibrillators by a US airline. N Engl J Med 2000;343:1210–6.
8. Caffrey SL, Willoughby PJ, Pepe PE, et al. Public use of automated external defibrillators. N Engl J Med 2002;347:1242–7.
9. Valenzuela TD, Roe DJ, Nichol G, et al. Outcomes of rapid defibrillation by security officers after cardiac arrest in casinos. N Engl J Med 2000;343:1206–9.
10. Eckstein M. The Los Angeles public access defibrillator (PAD) program: ten years after. Resuscitation 2012;83:1411–2.
11. The American Heart Association in collaboration with the International Liaison Committee on Resuscitation. Guidelines 2000 for cardiopulmonary resuscitation and emergency cardiovascular care, part 4: the automated external defibrillator. Key link in the chain of survival. Circulation 2000;102(Suppl 8): 160–76.
12. Maron BJ, Doerer JJ, Haas TS, et al. Sudden deaths in young competitive athletes: analysis of 1866 deaths in the United States, 1980–2006. Circulation 2009;119(8):1085–92.
13. Maron BJ. Sudden death in young athletes. N Engl J Med 2003;349(11):1064–75.
14. Corrado D, Basso C, Rizzoli G, et al. Does sports activity enhance the risk of sudden death in adolescents and young adults? J Am Coll Cardiol 2003; 42(11):1959–63.
15. Baggish AL, Hutter AM, Wang F, et al. Cardiovascular screening in college athletes with and without electrocardiography: a cross-sectional study. Ann Intern Med 2010;152:269–75.

16. Fuller CM, McNulty CM, Spring DA, et al. Prospective screening of 5,615 high school athletes for risk of sudden cardiac death. Med Sci Sports Exerc 1997;29:1131–8.

17. Wilson MG, Basavarajaiah S, Whyte GP, et al. Efficacy of personal symptom and family history questionnaires when screening for inherited cardiac pathologies: the role of electrocardiography. Br J Sports Med 2008;42:207–11.

18. Bessem B, Groot FP, Nieuwland W. The Lausanne recommendations: a Dutch experience. Br J Sports Med 2009;43:708–15.

19. Hevia AC, Fernández MM, Palacio JM, et al. ECG as a part of the preparticipation screening programme: an old and still present international dilemma. Br J Sports Med 2011;45:776–9.

20. Maron BJ, Thompson PD, Ackerman MJ, et al. Recommendations and considerations related to preparticipation screening for cardiovascular abnormalities in competitive athletes: 2007 update: a scientific statement from the American Heart Association. Circulation 2007;115:1643–55.

21. Drezner J, Corrado D. Is there evidence for recommending electrocardiogram as part of the preparticipation examination? Clin J Sport Med 2011; 21:18–24.

22. Marijon E, Tafflet M, Celermajer DS, et al. Sports-related sudden death in the general population. Circulation 2011;124(6):672–81.

23. Corrado D, Basso C, Pavei A, et al. Trends in sudden cardiovascular death in young competitive athletes after implementation of a preparticipation screening program. JAMA 2006;296(13):1593–601.

24. Maron BJ, Gohman TE, Aeppli D. Prevalence of sudden cardiac death during competitive sports activities in Minnesota high school athletes. J Am Coll Cardiol 1998;32:1881–4.

25. Van Camp SP, Bloor CM, Mueller FO, et al. Nontraumatic sports death in high school and college athletes. Med Sci Sports Exerc 1995;27:641–7.

26. Eckart RE, Shry EA, Burke AP, et al, Department of Defense Cardiovascular Death Registry Group. Sudden death in young adults—an autopsy-based series of a population undergoing active surveillance. J Am Coll Cardiol 2011;58(12):1254–61.

27. Atkins DL, Everson-Stewart S, Sears GK, et al. Epidemiology and outcomes from out-of-hospital cardiac arrest in children: the resuscitation outcomes consortium epistry—cardiac arrest. Circulation 2009;119:1484–91.

28. Meyer L, Stubbs B, Fahrenbruch C, et al. Incidence, etiology, and survival trends from cardiovascular-related sudden cardiac arrest in children and young adults ages 0–35: a 30-year review. Circulation 2012;126:1363–72.

29. Harmon KG, Asif IM, Klossner D, et al. Incidence of sudden cardiac death in national collegiate athletic association athletes. Circulation 2011;123(15): 1594–600.

30. Solberg EE, Gjertsen F, Haugstad E, et al. Sudden death in sports among young adults in Norway. Eur J Cardiovasc Prev Rehabil 2010;17(3):337–41.

31. Eckart RE, Scoville SL, Campbell CL, et al. Sudden death in young adults: a 25-year review of autopsies in military recruits. Ann Intern Med 2004;141(11):829–34.

32. Steinvil A, Chundadze T, Zeltser D, et al. Mandatory electrocardiographic screening of athletes to reduce their risk for sudden death proven fact or wishful thinking? J Am Coll Cardiol 2011;57(11):1291–6.

33. Drezner JA, Rao AL, Heistand J, et al. Effectiveness of emergency response planning for sudden cardiac arrest in United States high schools with automated external defibrillators. Circulation 2009; 120(6):518–25.

34. Drezner JA. ECG screening in athletes: time to develop infrastructure. Heart Rhythm 2011;8(10):1560–1.

35. Marek J, Bufalino V, Davis J, et al. Feasibility and findings of large-scale electrocardiographic screening in young adults: data from 32,561 subjects. Heart Rhythm 2011;8(10):1555–9.

36. Ljungqvist A, Jenoure PJ, Engebretsen L, et al. The International Olympic Committee (IOC) consensus statement on periodic health evaluation of elite athletes, March 2009. Clin J Sport Med 2009;19:347–65.

37. Corrado D, Pelliccia A, Bjørnstad HH, et al. Cardiovascular pre-participation screening of young competitive athletes for prevention of sudden death: proposal for a common European protocol. Consensus statement of the Study Group of Sport Cardiology of the Working Group of Cardiac Rehabilitation and Exercise Physiology and the Working Group of Myocardial and Pericardial Diseases of the European Society of Cardiology. Eur Heart J 2005; 26:516–24.

38. Dvorak J, Grimm K, Schmied C, et al. Development and implementation of a standardized precompetition medical assessment of international elite football players—2006 FIFA World Cup Germany. Clin J Sport Med 2009;19:316–21.

39. Pelliccia A. The preparticipation cardiovascular screening of competitive athletes: is it time to change the customary clinical practice? Eur Heart J 2007;28(22):2703–5.

40. Asif IA, Drezner JA. Sudden cardiac death and preparticipation screening: the debate continues—in support of electrocardiogram-inclusive preparticipation screening. Prog Cardiovasc Dis 2012;54(5): 445–50.

41. Maron BJ, Shirani J, Poliac LC, et al. Sudden death in young competitive athletes: clinical, demographic and pathological profiles. JAMA 1996;276:199–204.

42. Corrado D, Biffi A, Basso C, et al. 12-lead ECG in the athlete: physiological versus pathological abnormalities. Br J Sports Med 2009;43(9):669–76.

43. Corrado D, Pelliccia A, Heidbuchel H, et al, Section of Sports Cardiology, European Association of Cardiovascular Prevention and Rehabilitation. Recommendations for interpretation of 12-lead electrocardiogram in the athlete. Eur Heart J 2010;31(2):243–59.

44. Drezner JA, Asif IM, Owens DS, et al. Accuracy of ECG interpretation in competitive athletes: the impact of using standised ECG criteria. Br J Sports Med 2012;46(5):335–40.

45. Basso C, Maron BJ, Corrado D, et al. Clinical profile of congenital coronary artery anomalies with origin from the wrong aortic sinus leading to sudden death in young competitive athletes. J Am Coll Cardiol 2000;35(6):1493–501.

46. Varon J, Sternbach GL, Marik PE, et al. Automated external defibrillators: lessons from the past, present, and future. Resuscitation 1999;41:219–23.

47. Valenzuela TD, Roe DJ, Cretin S, et al. Estimating effectiveness of cardiac arrest interventions: a logistic regression survival model. Circulation 1997;96:3308–13.

48. Swor RA, Jackson RE, Cynar M, et al. Bystander CPR, ventricular fibrillation, and survival in witnessed, unmonitored out-of-hospital cardiac arrest. Ann Emerg Med 1995;25(6):780–4.

49. Link MS, Atkins DL, Passman RS, et al. Part 6: electrical therapies: automated external defibrillators, defibrillation, cardioversion, and pacing: 2010 American Heart Association Guidelines for Cardiopulmonary Resuscitation and Emergency Cardiovascular Care. Circulation 2010;122:S706–19.

50. Cummins RO, Eisenberg MS, Halstrom AP, et al. Survival of out-of-hospital cardiac arrest with early initiation of cardiopulmonary resuscitation. Am J Emerg Med 1985;3:114–9.

51. Cobb LA, Fahrenbruch CE, Walsh TR, et al. Influence of cardiopulmonary resuscitation prior to defibrillation in patients with out-of-hospital ventricular fibrillation. JAMA 1999;281:1182–8.

52. Waalweijn RA, Tijssen JG, Koster RW. Bystander initiated actions in out-of-hospital cardiopulmonary resuscitation: results from the Amsterdam Resuscitation Study (ARRESUST). Resuscitation 2001;50:273–9.

53. Larsen MP, Eisenberg MS, Cummins RO, et al. Predicting survival from out-of-hospital cardiac arrest: a graphic model. Ann Emerg Med 1993;22:1652–8.

54. Holmberg M, Holmberg S, Herlitz J. Incidence, duration, and survival of ventricular fibrillation, in out-of-hospital cardiac arrest patients in Sweden. Resuscitation 2000;44:7–17.

55. Chan PS, Krumholtz MH, Nichol G, et al. Delayed time to defibrillation after in-hospital cardiac arrest. N Engl J Med 2008;358:9–17.

56. Winkle RA. The effectiveness and cost effectiveness of public-access defibrillation. Clin Cardiol 2010; 33(7):396–9.

57. Drezner JA, Rogers KJ. Sudden cardiac arrest in intercollegiate athletes: detailed analysis and outcomes of resuscitation in nine cases. Heart Rhythm 2006;3(7):755–9.

58. Drezner JA, Toresdahl BG, Rao AL, et al. Outcomes from cardiac arrest in US high schools: a 2-year prospective study from the National Registry for AED Use in Sports. in press.

59. Andersen J, Courson RW, Kleiner DM, et al. National Athletic Trainers' Association position statement: emergency planning in athletics. J Athl Train 2002; 37:99–104.

60. Hazinski MF, Markenson D, Neish S, et al. Response to cardiac arrest and selected life-threatening medical emergencies: the medical emergency response plan for schools: a statement for healthcare providers, policymakers, school administrators, and community leaders. Circulation 2004; 109:278–91.

61. Myerburg RJ, Estes NA 3rd, Fontaine JM, et al. Task Force 10: automated external defibrillators. J Am Coll Cardiol 2005;45:1369–71.

62. Drezner JA, Courson RW, Roberts WO, et al. Inter-association task force recommendations on emergency preparedness and management of sudden cardiac arrest in high school and college athletic programs: a consensus statement. Clin J Sport Med 2007;17:87–103.

63. Berg RA, Hemphill R, Abella BS, et al. Part 5: adult basic life support: 2010 American Heart Association guidelines for cardiopulmonary resuscitation and emergency cardiovascular care. Circulation 2010; 122(18 Suppl 3):S685–705.

64. Sayre MR, Koster RW, Botha M, et al. Part 5: adult basic life support: 2010 international consensus on cardiopulmonary resuscitation and emergency cardiovascular care science with treatment recommendations. Circulation 2010;122: S298–324.

65. Bobrow BJ, Clark LL, Ewy GA, et al. Minimally interrupted cardiac resuscitation by emergency medical services for out-of-hospital cardiac arrest. JAMA 2008;299:1158–65.

66. Rea TD, Helbock M, Perry S, et al. Increasing use of cardiopulmonary resuscitation during out-of-hospital ventricular fibrillation arrest: survival implications of guideline changes. Circulation 2006;114: 2760–5.

67. Chi JS, Kloner RA. Stress and myocardial infarction. Heart 2003;89:475–6.

68. Wilbert-Lampen U, Leistner D, Greven S, et al. Cardiovascular events during World Cup soccer. N Engl J Med 2008;358:475–83.

69. Drezner JA, Rogers KJ, Zimmer RR, et al. Use of automated external defibrillators at NCAA division I universities. Med Sci Sports Exerc 2005;37(9):1487–92.

70. Borjesson M, Dugmore D, Mellwig KP, et al, Sports Cardiology Section of the European Association of Cardiovascular Prevention and Rehabilitation, European Society of Cardiology. Time for action regarding cardiovascular emergency care at sports arenas: a lesson from the Arena study. Eur Heart J 2010;31(12):1438–41.

71. Rothmier JD, Drezner JA, Harmon KG. Automated external defibrillators in Washington State high schools. Br J Sports Med 2007;41(5):301–5.

72. FIFA press release (5/28/2012) on AED's on every pitch. Available at: http://www.fifa.com/aboutfifa/organisation/bodies/congress/news/newsid=1637723/index.html.

73. National Conference on State Legislatures. State laws on cardiac arrest and defibrillators. Available at: http://www.ncsl.org/issues-research/health/laws-on-cardiac-arrest-and-defibrillators-aeds.aspx. Accessed September 1, 2012.

74. Jorgenson DB, Skarr T, Russell JK, et al. AED use in business, public facilities and homes by minimally trained first responders. Resuscitation 2003;59(2):225–33.

75. Schober P, van Dehn FB, Bierens JJ, et al. Public access defibrillation: time to access the public. Ann Emerg Med 2011;58:240–7.

76. Sakai T, Iwami T, Kitamura T, et al. Effectiveness of the new 'Mobile AED Map' to find and retrieve an AED: a randomised controlled trial. Resuscitation 2011;82(1):69–73.

77. Kovic I, Lulic I. Mobile phone in chain of survival. Resuscitation 2011;82(6):776–9.

78. Chugh SS, Reinier K, Balaji S, et al. Population-based analysis of sudden death in children: the Oregon sudden unexpected death study. Heart Rhythm 2009;6(11):1618–22.

Cardiovascular Evaluation of Master Athletes and Middle-aged/Senior Individuals Engaged in Leisure-time Sport Activities

Mats Börjesson, MD, PhD[a,b,]*, Luc Vanhees, PhD[c,d]

KEYWORDS

• Senior athletes • Cardiac evaluation • Master athletes • Sports • Risk stratification

KEY POINTS

• Regular physical activity provides significant health benefits, and most middle-aged/senior individuals should be encouraged to increase their level of physical activity.
• Acute bouts of intense exercise are also associated with increased risk of sudden cardiac death in apparently healthy individuals with an underlying and unknown cardiac disease.
• The rationale for the evaluation of middle-aged/senior individuals is to ensure safe participation in leisure-time sports or even competitive sports, with the aim of maximizing the benefits while minimizing the risks of exercise in middle-aged/senior individuals.
• Proper cardiovascular evaluation of these individuals engaged in moderate to intense leisure-time physical activities or sporting activities should be based on identification of underlying cardiovascular disease, the extent of the evaluation being dependent on the intended level of physical activity as well as the individual risk profile, including the habitual level of exercise.

BACKGROUND

Regular physical activity (PA), aerobic exercise, and cardiovascular fitness are all associated with a decrease in all-cause and cardiovascular mortality in the population, through its effect on several of the main risk factors for cardiovascular disease (CVD), including insulin sensitivity, lipid profile, blood pressure, and overweight.[1–4] Exercise also has positive effects on endothelial dysfunction, autonomic balance, and blood coagulation.[5–7] Indeed, a physically active life does seem to predict subsequent cardiovascular health, 20 years later.[8] Hence, PA is regarded as an important tool for prevention and treatment of coronary artery disease (CAD) by both the American Heart Association (AHA)[9–11] and the European Society of Cardiology (ESC).[12–15] The importance of exercise intensity is more emphasized in the recent publications of ESC than in earlier recommendations.

Although we want our middle-aged/senior population to exercise more for preventive reasons on one hand, there is on the other hand a potential

Disclosure: No relevant disclosure from any of the authors.
a Åstrand Laboratory, Swedish School of Sports and Health Science (GIH), Lidingövägen 1, 114 86 Stockholm, Sweden; b Department of Cardiology, Karolinska University Hospital, Solna, 171 76 Stockholm, Sweden; c Department Rehabilitation Sciences, Biomedical Sciences, KULeuven, Tervuursevest 101, B1501, 3000 Leuven, Belgium; d Research Group Lifestyle and Health, Faculty of Health Care, University of Applied Sciences, Bolognalaan 101, 3584 CJ Utrecht, The Netherlands
* Corresponding author.
E-mail address: mats.borjesson@gih.se

cardiacEP.theclinics.com

increased risk with acute intense exercise. Acute bouts of high-intensity exercise may trigger cardiac events, particularly in patients with underlying coronary atherosclerosis, through activation of the sympathetic nervous system and by increasing circulating catecholamines, which in turn may increase the risk of platelet adhesion, atherosclerotic plaque rupture, as well as malignant arrhythmias.[16–18] Thus, vigorous exertion has been found to increase the risk of acute cardiovascular events 2 to 56 times, in different studies.[10] Conversely, habitual exercise may diminish this triggering effect of exercise on the risk of acute cardiac events including sudden cardiac death (SCD), both in apparently healthy individuals as well as in patients with established CAD.[19,20]

The risk-benefit ratio may differ in relation to the individual's risk profile, with sedentary individuals with underlying CAD being at greatest risk.[21] Specifically, the risk-benefit ratio for more intense exercise in the middle-aged/senior person may be different compared with the younger individual. Vigorous intensity activity may theoretically offer a more diseased patient less benefits and greater risks, compared with individuals with less underlying disease. Elderly generally do have higher levels of underlying disease and thus may experience more cardiac events with vigorous activity. For example, the Copenhagen study showed that individuals who start PA at the age of 50 to 65 years had a higher risk for death in the next 15 years than those who did not.[22] Similarly, men with hypertension doing vigorous exercise may have a higher risk than those doing light-intensity PA.[23] The proposed mechanisms include the presence of underlying disease in combination with vigorous activity, serving as trigger in risk individuals.

The risk-benefit ratio of PA may also be different for the middle-aged 50 to 65 year olds, compared with the oldest individuals (age>75 years). Many studies have supported the protective role of low to medium-intensity activity in the elderly, with more vigorous activity not offering any additional benefits. Consequently, walking four hours a week was associated with lower mortality, but only in individuals older than 75 years.[24] Studies showing greater effect of moderate-intensity PA for the senior population may partly be explained by the fact that a given level may be more vigorous for the elderly person.[25–27] It is therefore suggested to use self-assessed "relative intensity" of activity, instead of absolute intensity, for advice on exercise for senior individuals. However, few of the oldest senior individuals may have the desire to take part in leisure-time sports anyway because of such barriers to exercise as lack of motivation, concomitant disease, and musculoskeletal disabilities.

Considering the potentially increased risk of cardiac events and SCD during PA in middle-aged/senior individuals with increased cardiovascular risk/disease, it is important to medically evaluate these individuals before their engagement in regular PA and leisure-time sports. The primary aim of such a medical evaluation is to ensure the safe participation in exercise, to achieve the maximal benefits of increased exercise while minimizing the risks. In addition, such an evaluation will give information (eg, fitness) that could be used in providing tailored information on the most suitable type and intensity of exercise (exercise prescription). The evaluation must also take into consideration possible barriers to exercise.

In this article, the authors review the existing recommendations regarding cardiovascular evaluation of athletes, focusing on master athletes and middle-aged/senior individuals, with or without known CAD, aiming for leisure-time sporting activities.

EXISTING RECOMMENDATIONS ON CARDIOVASCULAR EVALUATION OF ATHLETES
Screening of Young Competitive Athletes

In Europe (ESC) and in the United States (AHA), recommendations for cardiovascular preparticipation evaluation in young (<35 years old) competitive athletes have been previously published[28,29] and are widely implemented in the sporting community, for example by the FIFA and UEFA. These recommendations are not applicable in middle-aged/senior leisure-time athletes, because of markedly different causes of SCD in the younger and elderly athletic population. In the younger athletes, congenital/inherited cardiac diseases, most often hypertrophic cardiomyopathy, are the main causes of SCD, whereas in older athletes the most cases of SCD (>80%) are caused by underlying (silent/symptomatic) CAD.[10,30] In addition, competitive athletes, with an underlying cardiovascular abnormality, seem to have a higher risk of SCD, compared with nonathletes.[31] The recommendations on younger competitive athletes are also for this reason not applicable for use in senior/middle-aged leisure-time individuals.

Screening of Master Athletes

A paper from the AHA science advisory committee recommends preparticipation screening for all master athletes (defined as >40 years old and participating in competitive events).[32] The recommended cardiovascular evaluation consists of history and physical examination and also includes a routine standard 12-lead electrocardiogram (ECG). In addition, it is recommended that master athletes, having a moderate-to-high cardiovascular risk profile for CAD and desiring to enter vigorous master competitions, undergo symptom-limited maximal ECG exercise testing (treadmill or cycle ergometer). This cardiovascular risk profile includes all men older than 40 years and all women older than 50 years, with one additional coronary risk factor (hyperlipidemia, hypertension, smoking, diabetes mellitus/insulin resistance, or a positive family history) as well as all master athletes with symptoms suggestive of underlying CAD and all participants older than 65 years, regardless of symptoms or risk factors.

It should be clear that these recommendations are aimed for middle-aged/senior athletes, engaged in vigorous, competitive sporting activities and are not focused on individuals engaged or willing to engage in leisure-time sporting activities.

Screening at Health/fitness Facilities

Existing recommendations from the AHA/American College of Sports Medicine (ACSM) on cardiovascular screening of persons of all ages enlisting for training at health/fitness facilities were published in the late 1990s.[33] At that time 40% of the fitness facilities stated that they did not routinely use a screening interview or questionnaire to evaluate new members.[34] Importantly, 50% of health club/fitness facility members were older than 35 years, and the fastest growing group of users included those aged between 35 and 54 years and those who are older than 55 years.[33] Therefore, these recommendations have relevance for middle-aged/senior individuals willing to engage in leisure-time sports.

The AHA/ACSM propose to use self-administered screening questionnaires, such as the revised PA questionnaire (PAR-Q or the AHA preparticipation screening questionnaire),[35,36] to identify individuals with known CVD, symptoms of CVD, and/or risk factors for disease development, in need of further medical evaluation before starting an exercise program. After completion of the initial health appraisal and (when needed) the additional medical evaluation, participants are further classified into groups as follows: Class A (apparently healthy), Class B (presence of known, stable CVD with low risk for vigorous exercise), Class C (those at moderate to high risk for cardiac complications during exercise and/or who are unable to self-regulate activity), and Class D (unstable conditions with activity restrictions). This group classification may then be used to give advice on eligibility for

and intensity of exercise, suitable for each of these groups.

Recommendations for Participation in Leisure-time Exercise and Competitive Sports for Patients with CAD

These recommendations from the European Association of Cardiovascular Prevention and Rehabilitation (EACPR)[37] focus on the evaluation and eligibility for exercise and sports in patients with risk factors for and with established CAD. Individually prescribed leisure-time PA is advised and encouraged in patients with CAD for functional and preventive benefits. Competitive sports for these patients, however, may be contraindicated or restricted, depending on the probability of cardiac events and the demands of the sport, using the current classification into low-high static/low-high dynamic sports.[38]

The probability of cardiac events in patients with CAD may be divided into a lower risk and a higher risk group according to the results of the exercise test (exercise capacity, exercise-induced ischemia, arrhythmias during exercise), ejection fraction on echocardiography, the presence of any ventricular arrhythmias at rest, age, risk factors, and the result of coronary angiography (if performed).[37] In these recommendations, patients without evidence of CAD, but with one or more classical risk factors for CAD, may be classified as having a high-risk profile or a low-risk profile.

A *lower risk factor profile for developing a cardiovascular event* in individuals is defined as less than 5% 10-year risk according to Systematic Coronary Risk Evaluation (SCORE), without a history of diabetes mellitus or a positive family history for CAD, and a body mass index (BMI) less than 28 kg/m^2. The SCORE system is recommended by the ESC and is derived from large prospective studies.[39,40] The absolute risk of atherosclerotic cardiovascular death within 10 years is estimated based on a combination of physical examination and blood testing (age, sex, blood pressure, cholesterol, and smoking).

The higher risk factor profile for developing a fatal cardiovascular event is defined as (1 of the following 4) (1) the presence of various multiple risk factors, resulting in a 10-year risk greater than 5% now, or if extrapolated to 60 years of age in the SCORE chart; (2) markedly raised levels of total cholesterol (>8 mmol/L = 320 mg/dL) and LDL cholesterol (>6 mmol/L = 240 mg/dL) or blood pressure greater than 180/110 mm Hg; (3) diabetes mellitus type 2 or type 1 with microalbuminuria; and (4) individuals with a strong family history of premature CVD in first degree relatives younger than 50 years, as well as individuals with a BMI greater than 28 kg/m^2.[37]

The recommendations state that patients with CAD and with a high risk for cardiac events are not eligible for competitive sports but can profit from individually prescribed leisure-time PA (LTPA); patients with CAD and with a lower probability of cardiac events as well as subjects without diagnosed CAD but with a positive exercise test and high-risk profile (SCORE > 5%) are eligible for low/moderate static and low dynamic sports and individually prescribed LTPA. Patients without CAD and a high-risk profile + a negative exercise test and those with a low-risk profile (SCORE < 5%) are allowed both LTPA and competitive sports with a few exceptions.

These recommendations, however, focus specifically on patients at risk of or with established CAD, giving recommendations on eligibility for different sports, but do not focus on recommendations for the apparently healthy individual willing to engage in LTPA or intense sporting activities.

Cardiovascular Evaluation of Middle-aged/Senior Individuals Engaged in Leisure-time Sport Activities

The last recommendations addressed in this article are the recent recommendations from EACPR regarding middle-aged or senior individuals willing to participate in competitive or recreational sporting activities.[41] Because the population addressed in these recommendations is the specific focus of this article, we will discuss these recommendations more in detail.

The rationale for these recommendations is that the extent of the cardiovascular evaluation needed in middle-aged/senior individuals before start of (leisure-time) sports depends on the individual risk profile, incorporating the habitual level of PA, as well as the intended level of PA in the risk profile.

Individual risk profile

Classical risk factors The individual risk profile may be estimated from the burden of the known classical cardiovascular risk factors and the current level of fitness or habitual PA undertaken by the individual.[4,41] The identification of risk factors for CAD can be achieved in several ways. The first line of risk evaluation recommended is self-assessment (by the individual or by nonphysician health professionals), using validated questionnaires such as the AHA-preparticipation questionnaire[35] or the PAR-Q.[36]

This method of self-assessment could be used easily for large groups of individuals, thereby minimizing obstacles toward exercise.

In addition, more thorough risk assessment of the middle-aged/senior individual could be performed by a qualified physician, using the ESC Risk SCORE,[39] as described ealier.[41] In addition to the SCORE system, consideration should be given to additional major risk factors.[37]

Assessment of habitual PA/fitness In addition to using the traditional risk factors to assess the total risk profile of the middle-aged/senior individual, assessment of the habitual level of PA and/or fitness, are recommended. Although no ideal measure of PA exists, the level of PA could be assessed by several methods, including pedometers, accelerometers, and questionnaires,[42,43] the total volume of PA being a function of intensity (metabolic equivalent of tasks [METs]), duration (hours), and frequency. One MET is the intensity that equals the resting metabolic state of 3.5 mL 02/kg x minute, and the MET-values for different physical activities have previously been approximated.[44] The total volume of habitual PA, measured as MET-hours/week has been shown to discriminate individuals with low and high physical fitness level.[45]

An individual's fitness level may offer additional information to the risk assessed by the SCORE system (or similar scoring systems), identifying those individuals (physically inactive/low fitness) at higher risk.[46] Simple field test procedures such as the Cooper walk/run test or the Shuttle test[47] may be used to assess the individual aerobic capacity. The preferred test for assessment of the individual exercise capacity (fitness level) is maximal incremental exercise test, which provides clinically and prognostically important information.[43,48] Different submaximal exercise tests and field tests are instead commonly used outside the laboratory.[32]

Middle-aged/senior individuals may be categorized into 2 major groups according to their habitual PA level:

Sedentary individuals are defined as individuals who are not regularly engaged in PA or exercise, less than 2 MET-hours/week. This low-activity level has been associated with higher coronary event rates and a poorer prognosis. The recommendations[41] consider having a low cardiorespiratory fitness equivalent to having a high risk according to SCORE.

Active individuals are defined as individuals regularly engaged in leisure-time, even intense, noncompetitive sport activities, including master athletes.

The intended level of PA

The relative intensity of PA undertaken by the middle-aged/senior individual influences the burden on the cardiovascular system. Any categorization of the intensity of exercise as "moderate" or "vigorous" has to be related to the individual exercise tolerance rather than on absolute measures such as METs. For example, walking at a speed of 6 km/h may represent a vigorous, more than a low-moderate intensity of exercise for an obese individual with low fitness. To assess the relative intensity of exercise, simple tests such as the "Talk-test",[49] or more advanced laboratory tests such as heart-rate monitoring, could also be used.[43] Whatever method one chooses to use, obtaining an assessment of the individual cardiovascular fitness will aid the clinician, not only in risk stratification of obese individuals but also in making tailored prescription of exercise interventions possible. The physician will be able to prescribe a specific type of activity at the right level of (relative) intensity, based on the fitness level of the individual.

Different types of sports are classified according to the ESC classification[38] into 2 main categories: dynamic and static. Intensity is roughly divided into low, moderate, and high. High-intense exercise places considerable demands on the cardiovascular system, whereas lower-intensity exercise places a reduced demand on the heart. Individuals are stratified in 3 groups based on the relative intensity of intended PA, assessed by the individual or by a nonphysician:

1. Low-intensity intended PA, corresponding to 1,8 to 2,9 METs
2. Moderate-intensity intended PA, corresponding to 3 to 6 METs
3. High-intensity intended PA, including individuals participating/willing to participate in masters events such as long-distance cycling, city marathons, long-distance cross-country skiing, and triathlons, corresponding to more than 6 METs.

Recommendations

Based on the individual risk profile and the type/intensity of intended PA, the following levels of cardiovascular evaluation are recommended as appropriate for sedentary senior individuals and physically active middle-aged/senior individuals (which includes master athletes), respectively (**Figs. 1** and **2**).

Evaluation of sedentary middle-aged/senior individuals Apparently healthy middle-aged/senior individuals who wish to engage in low-intensity PA (<3 METs) are considered eligible for low-intensity PA without further evaluation, if the result of assessment of risk using validated self-assessed questionnaires is negative (see earlier) (see **Fig. 1**). The rationale for this choice is that we must not put unnecessary obstacles for exercise participation in middle-aged/senior individuals.

Middle-aged sedentary individuals, with a positive self-assessment, are advised to undergo additional thorough evaluation by a qualified physician, including reassessment of personal and family history, cardiovascular risk SCORE, physical examination, and a resting 12-lead ECG. The physical examination should include checks for Marfan syndrome, heart auscultation, and blood pressure in both arms and femoral/peripheral pulses.

Sedentary middle-aged/senior individuals should also have a maximal exercise test as part of the physician's evaluation before engaging in regular medium to high-intensity exercise (>3 METs), because they are defined as having a "higher risk factor profile" according to existing recommendations.[37,41] If the physician-led evaluation, including the exercise test, produces negative result, the individual is eligible for moderate or even high-intensity exercise training, but the authors recommend that cardiovascular evaluation is repeated on an individual basis. If the exercise test is abnormal (eg, showing inducible ischemia, malignant arrhythmias, or pathologic blood pressure response or decreased physical capacity), further proper evaluation by a cardiologist is necessary. Eligibility for further sports participation in case of confirmed CVD is advocated according to existing ESC recommendations.[38]

Evaluation of physically active middle-aged/senior individuals Physically active individuals have a statistically lower risk for cardiovascular complications during exertion compared with sedentary individuals (see **Fig. 2**). Active individuals, older than 35 years, who are already engaged in low-intensity activity and are asymptomatic, do not require cardiovascular evaluation, unless there is development of symptoms such as exertional syncope or chest pain or unexplained reduction in physical fitness.[50]

Physically active individuals of the same age, willing to participate in moderate-intensity (3–6 METs) PA, or continue being active at that level, should be evaluated by self-assessment questionnaires, as described earlier. Individuals with symptoms or history of CVD, derived from self-assessed questionnaire, should be evaluated by a physician including reassessment of the personal and family history, physical examination, risk SCORE, and 12-lead resting ECG.

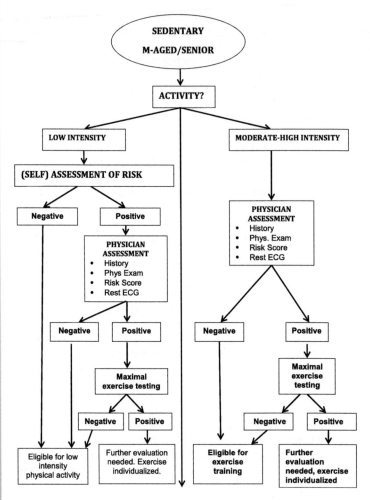

Fig. 1. Schematic presentation of the recommended cardiovascular evaluation of sedentary middle-aged/senior individuals willing to be engaged in leisure-time sport activities. (*Adapted from* Borjesson M, Urhausen A, Kouidi E, et al. Cardiovascular evaluation of middle-aged/senior individuals engaged in leisure-time sport activities: position stand from the sections of exercise physiology and sports cardiology of the European Association of Cardiovascular Prevention and Rehabilitation. Eur J Cardiovasc Prev Rehabil 2011;18:446–58; with permission.)

All physically active individuals older than 35 years contemplating or engaged in high-intensity (>6 METS) activity are subject to the same detailed evaluation by a qualified physician even in the absence of symptoms or other known risk factors for CAD. If positive, these individuals should undergo additional maximal exercise testing. Subjects are eligible for moderate/high-intensity exercise training if the exercise test is normal.

The patients may have associated comorbidities that could affect the possibility to reach an adequate level of activity, including orthopedic problems.[51] In addition, the use of medication could affect the ability to reach maximal pulse (beta-blockers, diuretics).[52] In the event of a positive exercise test, further evaluation is necessary to confirm/refute the presence of CAD or another cardiovascular abnormality. A reassessment of the risk factor profile, on an individual basis, is also recommended. The exercise test is important to aid the prescription of PA at the optimal intensity

for each individual. Regular reassessment of the cardiorespiratory fitness level, by a suitable evaluation method, should be part of the regular follow-up of these individuals.

DISCUSSION

In this article, the authors review existing recommendations/statements on screening from the United States and Europe. Most articles address screening procedures in young competitive athletes, with some similarities and discrepancies between United States and European recommendations reported.[29] However, the authors focus on older (>35 years of age) individuals, engaged in competitive sports (master athletes) or engaged or willing to engage in leisure-time sporting activities (LTPA). The reason for this focus is that more and more people older than 35 years are engaged in formalized or intense leisure-time exercise and sporting activities, although this is

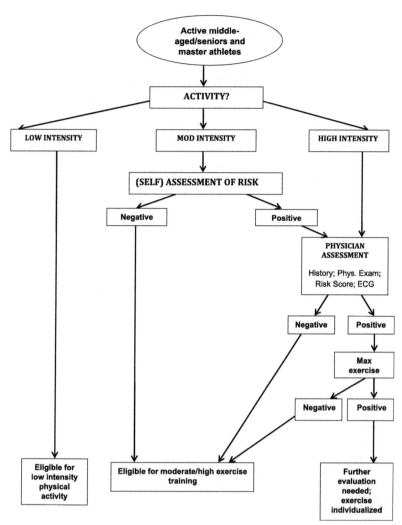

Fig. 2. Schematic presentation of the recommended cardiovascular evaluation of active middle-aged/senior individuals, including master athletes, engaged in leisure-time sport activities. (*Adapted from* Borjesson M, Urhausen A, Kouidi E, et al. Cardiovascular evaluation of middle-aged/senior individuals engaged in leisure-time sport activities: position stand from the sections of exercise physiology and sports cardiology of the European Association of Cardiovascular Prevention and Rehabilitation. Eur J Cardiovasc Prev Rehabil 2011;18:446–58; with permission.)

not necessarily accompanied by an increase in everyday PA of the individual. In fact, although more people are affiliated to a fitness facility or a sporting club, the overall activity level of the population seems to have decreased in recent years.

As a consequence, lifestyle-related diseases including obesity and diabetes mellitus are increasing worldwide, and fitness levels are decreasing. Similarly, while the number of participants in long-run races has increased exponentially, the average running time has increased, even after adjustment for age.[53] This trend may be even more pronounced in the future, potentially leading to an increasing number of middle-aged/

senior individuals wanting to take up sports, although having a worse risk factor profile, than previous generations.

Although regular PA provides significant health benefits and most middle-aged/senior individuals should be encouraged to increase their level of PA, this may also confer some increased risks. The well-known paradox of exercise says that, although regular exercise is associated with health benefits, acute exercise may be associated with increased risk of SCD, also in apparently healthy individuals, who may have an underlying silent cardiac disease. The risk-benefit ratio for each individual is the key. Proper recommendations for the evaluation of middle-aged/senior leisure-time athletes are important to gain the benefits of exercise at the minimum risks. In view of the well-known cardiovascular, morphologic, and metabolic benefits of regular PA, it is important to state that this evaluation in itself must not constitute a barrier for exercising, as the main goal is to increase the overall level of exercise, including leisure-time activity, safely in the middle-aged/senior population.

The US recommendations of evaluation of master athletes, encompassing only competitive athletes, advocate mandatory preparticipation evaluation (history and physical examination) of all master athletes and maximal exercise testing of all men aged more than 40 years (women > 50) with one additional risk factor and those with symptoms as well as all master athletes older than 65 years of age, regardless of risk factors or symptoms.[32]

Other recommendations from the AHA/ACSM are aimed at cardiovascular screening methods for persons of all ages, who are enlisting for training at health/fitness facilities.[33] They stratify individuals according to different risk categories and formulate suitable advice on eligibility for and intensity of exercise for each risk group. In these US recommendations, the fitness level or habitual level of PA or exercise is not considered part of the risk stratification process, although lack of exercise or a low aerobic capacity are considered to constitute major independent risk factors. Likewise, further evaluation by the physician is needed for final risk stratification in all instances when cardiovascular risk profile turns out to be increased at the preliminary self-assessment.

Finally, the authors have reported extensively on the recent EACPR recommendations,[19,23] because they were aimed at screening adult/senior active or sedentary individuals (willing to be) engaged in exercise/leisure-time PA/sports activities. These recommendations apply to individuals with a varying degree of cardiovascular risk profile and do selectively recommend thorough medical evaluation in individuals with higher risk of CAD according to SCORE.[37] The EACPR recommendations[41] specifically focused on apparently healthy individuals older than 35 years of age and proposed in their recommendations, in the assessment of the individual risk profile, also to consider the habitual and intended level of exercise/sporting activity. These screening recommendations target the population of older individuals and provide a practical solution for facilitating safe exercise prescription and sports participation in middle-aged/senior individuals.

SUMMARY

Regular PA provides significant health benefits and most middle-aged/senior individuals should therefore be encouraged to increase their level of PA. On the other hand, acute bouts of intense exercise are also associated with increased risk of SCD in apparently healthy individuals with an underlying and unknown cardiac disease. The risk-benefit ratio for each individual may look different, depending on the individual risk profile. The rationale for the evaluation of middle-aged/senior individuals is to ensure the safe participation in leisure-time sports or even competitive sports, with the aim of maximizing the benefits while minimizing the risks of exercise in this group.

Proper cardiovascular evaluation of these individuals engaged or willing to engage in moderate to intense leisure-time PA or sporting activities should be based on identification of underlying CVD, the extent of the evaluation being dependent on the intended level of PA, as well as the individual risk profile, including the habitual level of exercise.

REFERENCES

1. Iestra JA, Kromhout D, van der Schouw YT, et al. Effect size estimates of lifestyle and dietary changes on all-cause mortality in coronary artery disease patients: a systematic review. Circulation 2005;112: 924–34.
2. Blair SN, Kohl HW, Paffenbarger RS Jr, et al. Physical fitness and all-cause mortality: a prospective study of healthy men and women. JAMA 1989;262: 2395–401.
3. Paffenbarger RS Jr, Hyde RT, Wing AL, et al. The association of changes in physical activity and other lifestyle characteristics with mortality among men. N Engl J Med 1993;328:538–45.
4. Kodama S, Kazumi S, Tanaka S, et al. Cardiorespiratory fitness as quantitative predictor of all-cause mortality and cardiovascular events in healthy men and women. A meta-analysis. JAMA 2009;301: 2024–35.
5. Hambrecht R, Wolf A, Gielen S, et al. Effect of exercise on coronary endothelial function in patients with coronary artery disease. N Engl J Med 2000;342: 454–60.
6. Panagiotakos DB, Kokkinos P, Manios Y, et al. Physical activity and markers of inflammation and thrombosis related to coronary artery disease. Prev Cardiol 2004;7:190–4.
7. Yarnell JW, Sweetnam PM, Rumley A, et al. Lifestyle and hemostatic risk factors for IHD: the Caerphilly study. Arterioscler Thromb Vasc Biol 2000;20:271–9.

8. Gulsvik AK, Thelle DS, Samuelson SO, et al. Ageing, physical activity and mortality-a 42 year follow-up study. Int J Epidemiol 2011;41:521–30.

9. Thompson PD, Buchner D, Pina IL, et al. AHA scientific statement: exercise and physical activity in the prevention and treatment of atherosclerotic cardiovascular disease. Circulation 2003;107:3109–16.

10. Thompson PD, Franklin BA, Balady GJ, et al. Exercise and acute cardiovascular events. Placing the risks into perspective. A scientific statement from the American heart Association Council on nutrition, physical activity, and metabolism and the Council on Clinical Cardiology. Circulation 2007; 115:2358–68.

11. Williams MA, Haskell WL, Ades PA, et al, American Heart Association Council on Clinical Cardiology, American Heart Association Council on Nutrition, Physical Activity and Metabolism. Resistance exercise in individuals with and without cardiovascular disease: 2007 update. Circulation 2007;116:572.

12. Perk J, deBacker G, Gohlke H, et al. European Guidelines on cardiovascular disease prevention in clinical practice (version 2012): the fifth Joint Task Force of the European Society of Cardiology and other Societies on cardiovascular disease prevention in clinical practice. Eur Heart J 2012;33: 1635–701.

13. Vanhees L, DeSutter J, Geladas N, et al. Importance of characteristics and modalities of physical activity and exercise in the mangement of cardiovascular health within the general population: recommendations from the EACPR (part I). Eur J Prev Cardiol 2012;19:670–86.

14. Vanhees L, Geladas N, Hansen D, et al. Importance of characteristics and modalities of physical activity and exercise in the management of cardiovascular health in individuals with cardiovascular risk factors: recommendations from the EACPR (part II). Eur J Prev Cardiol 2012;19:1005–33.

15. Vanhees L, Rauch B, Piepoli M, et al. Importance of characteristics and modalities of physical activity and exercise in the management of cardiovascular health in individuals with cardiovascular disease (part III). Eur J Prev Cardiol 2012;19:1333–56.

16. Burke AP, Farb A, Malcolm GT, et al. Plaque rupture and sudden death related to exertion in men without coronary artery disease. JAMA 1999;281:921–6.

17. Peronnet F, Cleroux J, Perreault H, et al. Plasma norepinephrine response to exercise before and after training in humans. J Appl Physiol 1981;51: 812–5.

18. Willich SN, Lewis M, Lowel H, et al. Physical exertion as a trigger of acute myocardial infarction. N Engl J Med 1993;329:1684–90.

19. Mittleman MA, Maclure M, Tofler GH, et al. Triggering of acute myocardial infarction by heavy physical exertion. Protection against triggering by regular exertion. Determinants of Myocardial Onset Study Investigators. N Engl J Med 1993;329:1677–83.

20. Siskovick DS, Weiss NS, Fletcher RH, et al. Habitual vigorous exercise and primary cardiac arrest: effect of other risk factors on the relationship. J Chronic Dis 1984;37:625–31.

21. Maron BJ. The paradox of exercise. N Engl J Med 2000;343:1409–11.

22. Hein HO, Suadicani P, Sörensen H, et al. Changes in physical activity level and the risk of ischemic heart disease. Scand J Med Sci Sports 1994;4:57–64.

23. Shaper AG, Wannamethee SG, Walker M. Physical activity, hypertension and risk of heart attack in men without evidence of ischemic heart disease. J Hum Hypertens 1994;8:3–10.

24. Woodcock J, Franco OH, Orsini N, et al. Non-vigorous physical activity and all-cause mortality: a systematic review and meta-analysis report of cohort studies. Int J Cardiol 2011;40:121–38.

25. Bemborn O, vanderLaan M, Haight T, et al. Leisure-time physical activity and all-cause mortality in an elderly cohort. Epidemiology 2009;20:424–30.

26. Swain DP, Franklin BA. Comparison of cardiorespiratory benefits of vigorous versus moderate intensity aerobic activity. Am J Cardiol 2006;97:141–7.

27. Lee IM, Sesso HD, Oguma Y, et al. Relative intensity of physical activity and risk of coronary heart disease. Circulation 2003;107:1110–6.

28. Corrado D, Pelliccia A, Bjornstad HH, et al. Cardiovascular pre-participation screening of young competitive athletes for prevention of sudden death: proposal for a common European protocol. Eur Heart J 2005;26:516–24.

29. Pelliccia A, Zipes DP, Maron BJ. Bethesda Conference #36 and the European Society of Cardiology Consensus Recommendations revisited: a comparison of US and European criteria for eligibility and disqualification of competitive athletes with cardiovascular abnormalities. J Am Coll Cardiol 2008;52: 1990–6.

30. Corrado D, Basso C, Pavei A, et al. Trends in sudden cardiovascular death in young competitive athletes after implementation of a preparticipation screening program. JAMA 2006;296:1593–601.

31. Corrado D, Basso C, Rizzoli G, et al. Does sports activity enhance the risk of sudden death in adolescents and young adults? J Am Coll Cardiol 2003;42: 1964–6.

32. Maron BJ, Araujo CG, Thompson PD, et al. Recommendations for preparticipation screening and the assessment of cardiovascular disease in master athletes: an advisory for healthcare professionals from the working group pfs of the World Heart Federation, the International federation of Sports Medicine and the American Heart Association committe on Exercise, Cardiac rehabilitation and Prevention. Circulation 2001;103:327–34.

33. Balady GJ, Chaitman B, Driscoll D, et al. AHA/ACSM scientific statement: recommendations for cardiovascular screening, staffing, and Emergency policies at health/fitness facilities. Circulation 1998;97:2283–93.

34. McInnis KJ, Hayakawa S, Balady GJ. Cardiovascular screening and emergency procedures at health clubs and fitness centers. Am J Cardiol 1997;80:380–3.

35. Balady GJ, Larson MG, Vasan RS, et al. Usefulness of exercise testing in the prediction of coronary disease risk among asymptomatic persons as a function of the Framingham risk score. Circulation 2004;110:1920–5.

36. Thomas S, Reading J, Shephard RJ. Revision of the physical activity Readiness questionnaire (PAR-Q). Can J Sport Sci 1992;17:338–45.

37. Börjesson M, Assanelli D, Carré F, et al. ESC Study Group of Sports Cardiology: recommendations for participation in leisure-time physical activity and competitive sports for patients with iscaemic heart disease. Eur J Cardiovasc Prev Rehabil 2006;13:137–49.

38. Pelliccia A, Fagard R, Bjornstad H, et al. Recommendations for competitive sports participation in athletes with cardiovascular diseae: a consensus document from the Study Group of Sports Cardiology of the Working Group of Cardiac Rehabilitation and exercise Physiology and the Working Group of Myocardial and Pericardial diseases of the European Society of Cardiology. Eur Heart J 2005;26:1422–45.

39. Conroy RM, Pyörälä K, Fitzgerald AP, et al. Estimation of ten-year risk of fatal cardiovascular disease in Europe: the SCORE project. Eur Heart J 2003;24:987–1003.

40. Graham I, Atar D, Borch-Johnsen K, et al, European Society of Cardiology (ESC) Committee for Practice Guidelines (CPG). European guidelines on cardiovascular disease prevention in clinical practice: executive summary. Fourth Joint Task Force of the European Society of Cardiology and other Socities. Eur Heart J 2007;28:2375–414.

41. Borjesson M, Urhausen A, Kouidi E, et al. Cardiovascular evaluation of middle-aged/senior individuals engaged in leisure-time sport activities: position stand from the sections of exercise physiology and sports cardiology of the European Association of Cardiovascular Prevention and Rehabilitation. Eur J Cardiovasc Prev Rehabil 2011;18:446–58.

42. Warren JM, Ekelund U, Besson H, et al. Assessment of physical activity- a review of methodologies with reference to epidemiological research: a report of the exercise physiology setion of the European Association of Cardiovascular Prevention and Rehabilitation. Eur J Cardiovasc Prev Rehabil 2010;17:127–39.

43. Vanhees L, Lefevre J, Philippaerts R, et al. How to assess physical activity? How to assess physical fitness? Eur J Cardiovasc Prev Rehabil 2005;12:102–14.

44. Ainsworth BE, Haskell WL, Whitt MC, et al. Compendium of physical activities: an update of activity codes and MET intensities. Med Sci Sports Exerc 2000;32(Suppl):S498–504.

45. Saltin B. Physiological effects of physical conditioning. In: Hansen AT, Schnor P, Rose G, editors. Ischaemic heart disease: the strategy of postponement. Chicago: Year Book Medical Publishers; 1977. p. 104–15.

46. Laukkanen JA, Rauramaa R, Salonen JT, et al. The predictive value of cardiorespiratory fitness combined with coronary risk evaluation and the risk of cardiovascular and all-cause death. J Intern Med 2007;262:263–72.

47. Grants S, Corbett K, Amjad AM, et al. A comparison of methods of predicting maximum oxygen uptake. Br J Sports Med 1995;29:147–52.

48. Mezzani A, Agostini P, Cohen-Solal A, et al. Standards for the use of cardiopulmonary exercise testing for the functional evaluation of cardiac patients: a report from the exercise physiology section of the European association for cardiovascular prevention and rehabilitation. Eur J Cardiovasc Prev Rehabil 2009;16:249–67.

49. Vanhees L, Stevens A. Exercise intensity: a matter of measuring or of talking? J Cardiopulm Rehabil 2006;26:78–9.

50. Talbot LA, Morrell CH, Fleg JL, et al. Changes in leisure-time physical activity and risk of all-cause mortality in men and women: the Baltimore longitudinal study of aging. Prev Med 2007;45:169–76.

51. Anandacoomarasamy A, Fransen M, March L. Obesity and the musculoskeltal system. Curr Opin Rheumatol 2009;21:71–7.

52. Guidry MA, Blanchard BE, Thompson PD, et al. The influence of short and long duration beta-blockade on the blood pressure response to an acute bout of dynamic exercise. Am J Cardiol 2006;151:1322–7.

53. Aagaard P, Sahlén A, Braunschweig F. Performance trends and cardiac biomarkers in a 30-km cross-countr race 1993-2007. Med Sci Sports Exerc 2012;44:894–9.

Sudden Death in Marathon Runners

Jason James, BSc, Ahmed Merghani, MBBS,
Sanjay Sharma, MD*

KEYWORDS

- Endurance athlete • Exercise • Marathon running • Sudden cardiac arrest • Sudden cardiac death
- Screening

KEY POINTS

- The reported incidence of sudden death in marathons varies widely from 0.54 to 2.1/100,000.
- Death in marathon runners is frequently observed in the fifth and sixth decade of life, and most deaths occur in relatively experienced runners who have participated in previous marathons.
- A recent study showed that runners who suffered a sudden cardiac arrest due to hypertrophic cardiomyopathy were younger and less likely to survive compared with those with coronary artery disease.
- Cardiac diseases frequently implicated in sudden cardiac death during sport include coronary artery disease, hypertrophic cardiomyopathy, arrhythmogenic right ventricular cardiomyopathy, valvular disease, anomalous coronary arteries, coronary vasospasm, coronary dissection, myocardial bridging, and ion channelopathies, such as Brugada syndrome and long QT syndrome.
- Hyponatremia and exercise-related heatstroke are important causes of noncardiac sudden death in marathon runners.

INTRODUCTION

The benefits of exercise are well established. Active individuals have favorable lipid and blood pressure profiles and a 50% reduction in the risk of developing coronary artery disease (CAD).[1,2] In addition to the cardiovascular benefits, physical activity also confers benefits in the prevention of certain malignancies, treatment of mild depression, and potential retardation of dementia.[3] A meta-analysis of 27,100 participants followed for a mean duration of 12 years reported a 30% reduction in all-cause mortality in those who led a regularly active lifestyle consisting of exercise of moderate intensity.[4] Studies involving retired athletes have demonstrated a longevity benefit of around 6 years compared with sedentary counterparts.[5]

The Department of Health (UK) recommends 150 minutes of moderate exercise per week for adults, and 60 minutes per day for children.[6] Moderate intensity exercise is defined as a metabolic equivalent of 3 to 6, which can range from a brisk walk at 4 mph to cycling at 10 to 12 mph.[6] The American College of Sports Medicine also states that shorter periods of vigorous exercise (equivalent to jogging) can be performed for 20 minutes 3 times per week.[7]

These recommendations fall considerably short of the amount of training required to run a 26.2-mile marathon, which is a grueling endurance event associated with huge demands on the

Disclosures: Sanjay Sharma is the Medical Director of the London Marathon.
Department of Cardiovascular Sciences, St George's University of London, Cranmer Terrace, London SW17 0RE, UK
* Corresponding author. Department of Cardiology, St George's University of London, Cranmer Terrace, London SW17 0RE, UK.
E-mail address: ssharma21@hotmail.com

Card Electrophysiol Clin 5 (2013) 43–51
http://dx.doi.org/10.1016/j.ccep.2013.01.003

body's metabolism and musculoskeletal system. Most conditioned runners have coped well with the stresses of the marathon since its inception as an Olympic event in 1896 with tremendous improvements in performance since that time. Although the original marathon was completed in 2 hours, 58 minutes, and 50 seconds, by a Greek athlete, the Olympic Record has since been shortened to a staggering 2 hours, 6 minutes, and 32 seconds, set by Samuel Kamau Wanjiru of Kenya in 2008.[8]

In recent times, the number of marathons held and rates of participation have vastly expanded, with more than 500 marathons ran per year worldwide consisting of at least 1 million runners each year.[9] In 1981, the first London Marathon was held, with fewer than 7000 participants competing, which is less than 5 times than that of the race in 2012. These competitors range from elite athletes to amateur enthusiasts, all challenging the limits of human endurance.

The potential for the marathon to take its toll on vulnerable or predisposed participants dates back to 490 BC when the soldier Pheidippides died suddenly after reportedly running from Marathon to Athens (approximately 25 miles) to announce victory over the Persians in the Battle of Marathon.[8] Large marathons are frequently televised and emphasis is frequently placed on the extraordinary ability of the human being, the laudable nature of charity runners, and the strength and determination of participating individuals who have overcome malignancies and other life-threatening illnesses. However, it is also difficult to ignore the sight of multiple collapsed participants during such a broadcast, which underscores the physically destructive impact of the marathon on the human body. The occasional sudden death occurring during or after a race receives considerable media attention and has often called for marathons to be banned. The ensuing article focuses on the incidence of sudden death in marathons, the demographics of the victims, and the causes implicated.

EPIDEMIOLOGY
Incidence

The incidence of sudden death (SD) in marathons varies widely from 0.54 to 2.1/100,000 between reports (**Table 1**). Among the highest estimate was from Maron and colleagues,[10] who studied 215,413 marathon runners from the Marine Corps and Twin Cities marathons and reported an incidence of sudden death to be 2 per 100,000 (1 in 50,000).[10] A larger, more recent study by Kim and colleagues[15] estimated the incidence at 0.39/100,000 in a population of 10.9 million marathon runners. The considerable variation in numbers is likely due to differences in methodology and limitations of the various studies. Maron and colleagues[10] studied the rate of death in 2 marathons over 2 decades, compared with all marathons and half marathons run in the United States over a 10-year period studied by Kim and colleagues.[15] The data by Maron were predominantly collected from an accurate account maintained by the race directors. In contrast, approximately two-thirds of the cohort studied by Kim and colleagues were engaged in a half marathon and data relied on recall as well as electronic search engines. The likely main contributor to the lower reported incidence by Kim and colleagues[15] is the higher prevalence of half marathon runners who had a much lower incidence of cardiac arrest compared with full marathon runners (0.27 vs 1.01/100,000).

Table 1
The incidence of sudden death and cardiac arrest in the literature

Author	Year of Study	Sample Size	Events (n)	Death (D) Arrest (A)	Incidence/100,000
Maron et al,[10] 1996	1976–1994	215,413	4	D	2
Redelmeier and Greenwald,[11] 2007	1975–2005	3,292,268	26	D	0.8
Tunstall-Pedoe,[12] 2007	1981–2006	650,000	8	D	1.25
			14	A	2.15
Webner et al,[13] 2012	1976–2009	1,710,052	10	D	0.58
			30	A	1.75
Mathews et al,[14] 2012	2000–2009	3,718,336	28	D	0.75
Kim et al,[15] 2012	2000–2010	10,871,000	42	D	0.39
			59	A	0.54

Webner and colleagues[13] reported an incidence of 0.58/100,000 in American marathon runners (1 in 172,000 runners). However, this may have also been affected by recall bias since the data were derived from a voluntary web based survey conducted on medical directors of several marathons. The authors noted a limitation that medical directors may be more inclined to respond to the survey if they had experienced a successful resuscitation of a sudden cardiac arrest (SCA). Mathews and colleagues[14] reported an incidence of 0.75/100,000 among American marathon runners but the study was limited due to the inability to contact a proportion of the medical directors of the marathons studied and therefore placed reliance on the media. There are also inconsistencies regarding the time period in which a death was thought to be due to the race itself. Mathews and colleagues included deaths that occurred 24 hours after the race, whereas Kim and colleagues[15] only considered those who had an SCA within an hour of finishing the race.[14]

The London marathon is among the 5 largest marathons in the world and data relating to rates of cardiac arrest event and outcomes have been meticulously collated since the inception of the race in 1981. Detailed information following each death is provided because the medical director attends the autopsy examination and subsequent inquests. Among the 650,000 participants between 1981 and 2006, there were 14 SCAs, of which 8 were fatal, providing an incidence of 1.25/100,000.[12] In the past 6 years the London Marathon has witnessed another 4 SCAs, with 2 fatalities from exercise-associated hyponatremia (2007) and sudden arrhythmic death syndrome (2012), respectively, among an additional 210,000 runners, providing a rate of overall SCA of 2.1/100,000 (Sanjay Sharma, personal communication, 2012).

Demographics

Age

The age distribution of marathon runners is broad, ranging from teenagers to octogenarians. The most recent London marathon exemplifies this (**Fig. 1**), where the most prevalent ages were between 30 and 49 years old. Death in marathon runners is frequently observed in the fifth and sixth decade of life (**Table 2**). Most deaths occur in relatively experienced runners who have participated in previous marathons.[12,14,15] It is noteworthy that the age of death may be influenced by underlying cardiac pathologic abnormality. A recent study showed that runners who suffered a SCA due to hypertrophic cardiomyopathy were younger and less likely to survive compared with those with CAD.[15]

Roberts and colleagues[16] studied more than 500,000 marathon runners from 1982 to 2009 at the Twin Cities and Marine Corps marathons in the United States and noted that the population of marathon runners was aging. In 1982, the authors found that 25% of the men and 15% of the women were greater than 40 years of age. In contrast, these figures increased in 2009, to 45% and 29%, respectively,[16] implying that a greater proportion of marathon runners are moving into the higher risk age groups.

Gender

Marathon running has been historically dominated by men; however, the proportion of female marathon runners has increased significantly each year. Roberts and colleagues[16] observed an increase from 12% to 39% between 1982 and 2009. Data from the London Marathon show that even in the last 4 years there continues to be a steady increase in female participants (**Fig. 2**).

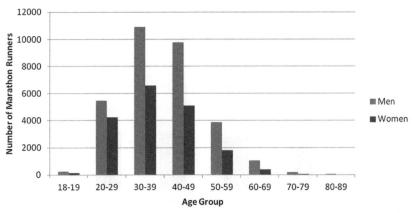

Fig. 1. Age distribution among runners of the London Marathon, 2012 (Sanjay Sharma, Medical Director of the London Marathon, unpublished data, 2012).

Table 2
Cardiovascular marathon events by age

Publication	Sudden Death		Survivor of Sudden Cardiac Arrest	
	N	Average Age	N	Average Age
Kim et al,[15] 2012	42	39	17	49
Mathews et al,[14] 2012	28	42[a]	N/A	N/A
Redelmeier and Greenwald,[11] 2007	21	41[b]	N/A	N/A
Tunstall-Pedoe,[12] 2007	8	48	6	48
Roberts et al,[16] 2012	7	44	7	48
Maron et al,[10] 1996	4	37	N/A	N/A
Cohen and Ellis,[17] 2012	2	53	1	63

Abbreviation: N/A, Not available.
[a] Refers to median average age, not mean age.
[b] Men only.

It has long been known that the risk of cardiovascular disease is more prevalent in men than in women, and male sex is considered a nonmodifiable risk factor. This pattern is also reflected in rates of SCA and SD in marathon runners, where male predominance is a ubiquitous finding. Recent studies by Kim and colleagues[15] and Mathews and colleagues[14] reported a male bias of 86% and 79%, respectively. In the London Marathon 13 of 14 SCAs affected men. The higher rate of participation among men (approximately 65%) does not explain the male majority completely, suggesting that male sex is an independent risk factor.

Trends in rates of sudden death

There has been a worrying increase in the incidence of SD in male marathon runners. The recent study by Kim and colleagues[15] observed a statistically significant rise in the latter half of the previous decade in male deaths (0.55 vs 1.17/100,000, $P = .02$). This finding is reiterated by a further study comparing male deaths between 1982–1999 and 2000–2009 (incidence 1.3/100,000 [95% CI 0.3–3.9] vs 2.0/100,000 [95% CI 0.4–5.8]).[16] Some authors have attributed this escalation to marathons being a free for all entrants, which may attract more high-risk men with occult cardiac disease.[15] Interestingly, the increase in rates of death in male runners has not been reflected in their female counterparts. Although female participation has more than tribled between 1982 and 2009, there have been no new fatalities in female runners in the time period 2000 to 2009. This is in contrast to the male incidence of 3.8/100,000 and 4.6/100,000 between 1982–2009 and 2000–2009, respectively.[16] One potential explanation for the sex discrepancy in rates of SGAs/sudden cardiac

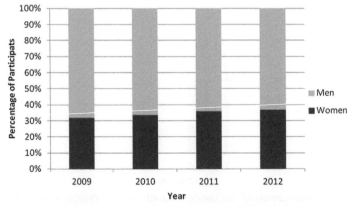

Fig. 2. Participation numbers divided by gender, London Marathon 2009–2012.

death (SCD) is that the high-risk age category for women is more than 50 and for men it is more than 35 for CAD. Therefore, as the age of marathon participation increases, a greater proportion of men enter higher risk groups, whereas women have more immunity at parallel ages.[16]

ETIOLOGY

Understanding the cause of SD in marathon runners is important in risk stratification, as well as adopting preventative strategies. Deaths may be broadly categorized into cardiac and non-cardiac causes (**Fig. 3**). For the purpose of this review, and the fact that cardiac pathologies are far more common, cardiac deaths are the primary focus. The most prevalent causes of SD in marathon runners are CAD and hypertrophic cardiomyopathy (HCM).[10,12,14,15] Noncardiac causes include exercise-associated hyponatremia (often caused by overhydration), cerebrovascular accidents, and heatstroke.

Cardiac Diseases

Cardiac diseases frequently implicated in SCD during sport include CAD, HCM, arrhythmogenic right ventricular cardiomyopathy, valvular disease, anomalous coronary arteries, coronary vasospasm, coronary dissection, myocardial bridging, and ion channelopathies, such as Brugada syndrome and long QT syndrome.

In a large retrospective analysis of all marathons and half marathons run in the United States during 2000 to 2009, complete clinical data were

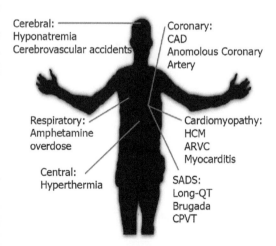

Cerebral:
Hyponatremia
Cerebrovascular accidents

Coronary:
CAD
Anomolous Coronary Artery

Respiratory:
Amphetamine overdose

Central:
Hyperthermia

Cardiomyopathy:
HCM
ARVC
Myocarditis

SADS:
Long-QT
Brugada
CPVT

Fig. 3. Cause of sudden death in marathon runners. ARVC, arrhythmogenic right ventricular cardiomyopathy; CAD, coronary artery disease; CPVT, catecholaminergic polymorphic ventricular tachycardia; HCM, hypertrophic cardiomyopathy; SADS, sudden arrhythmic death syndrome.

obtained for 31 of 59 SCAs (23 nonsurvivors and 8 survivors).[15] Most patients had HCM (n = 8) or possible HCM (n = 7). Hypertrophic cardiomyopathy was defined as a combination of increased cardiac mass with supportive findings, consisting of family history, characteristics of gross anatomic architecture, increased left ventricular wall thickness, and disease-specific histologic findings.[15] The criteria used to define "possible HCM" included increased left ventricular mass in the absence of some of the criteria mentioned earlier. The cause of the other 8 deaths were hyponatremia (n = 2), no evident abnormality on autopsy or presumed primary arrhythmia (n = 2), arrhythmogenic right ventricular cardiomyopathy (n = 1), unknown (n = 2), and hyperthermia (n = 1). Among the 8 survivors, CAD was the predominant cause of cardiac arrest (n = 5), with 3 runners having an 85% to 95% stenosis in a single vessel, 1 runner with 2-vessel disease, and 1 runner with triple-vessel disease. The other causes of SCA survivors were nonischemic ventricular tachycardia (n = 2) and unknown (n = 1).[15]

The key findings of the study mentioned above suggest that HCM is the leading cause of death in marathon running, accounting for approximately 65% of all deaths. Furthermore, CAD was not a main diagnosis in any of the fatalities in the study, but was featured in 63% of those who survived an SCA. The authors concluded that cardiac arrest from HCM has a far worse prognosis than CAD in respect to SCA in marathon runners.[15]

The observation that HCM is the commonest cause of death is not replicated in other studies. A study by Maron and colleagues[10] evaluating SCAs in more than 200,000 runners participating in the Twin Cities (1982–1994) and Marine Corps (1976–1994) marathons over a cumulative period of 30 years reported 4 SCDs. Of these, 75% were attributed to CAD (n = 3), and 1 death was attributed to anomalous coronary arteries. In a more elaborate study by Roberts and colleagues[16] who studied more than 500,000 participants (1982–2009) in the same marathons reported 14 SCAs (including 7 that were fatalities), 12 SCAs attributed to CAD. All 12 diagnoses of CAD were in men aged 39 and over (6 nonsurvivors, 6 survivors). The only SCD ascribed to another cause in a female fatality was due to anomalous coronary arteries, and the only survivor of an SCA in the absence of CAD was a 28-year-old man with mitochondrial myopathy.[16] Data from the London Marathon between 1981 and 2012 (Sanjay Sharma, personal communication, 2012) also suggest that CAD is the most common cause of SCA; of the 18 SCAs, 12 (66%) were due to CAD.

It is important to note that several runners with significant coronary disease at autopsy also revealed an increased cardiac mass,[15] which may have been a physiologic manifestation of athletic training. Therefore, it is possible that many of the athletes deemed to have died of "probable HCM" in the study by Kim and colleagues[15] may have died of other causes, such as ion channel diseases, electrolyte disturbances, and heat injury. Careful analysis of the autopsy data from the study showed that some athletes deemed to have died of probable and definite HCM also had significant CAD with luminal stenosis between 70% and 90%, suggesting that the contribution of CAD to the actual death is difficult to exclude even in the absence of obvious infarction. Indeed plaque rupture is an uncommon finding at autopsy in athletes who have extensive coronary atherosclerosis, suggesting that most die from ischemia-induced cardiac arrhythmias.[18]

The cause of SD in marathon runners is influenced by age. Deaths from HCM primarily affect relatively young runners, whereas deaths from CAD occur in runners who are on average 10 years older and predominate in men ≥50 years old. A prime example of this age segregation is from research conducted by Mathews and colleagues[14] between 2000 and 2009 in more than 3 million marathon runners in the United States. The authors collated 28 cases of SD, with 14 aged ≥45 years, and 14 aged less than 45 years. The diagnosis in 13 of 14 SCDs ≥45 years old was CAD, highlighting the increase in risk associated with increasing age. In stark contrast, none of the deceased runners less than 45 years showed significant CAD, but revealed other structural or congenital abnormalities, including HCM (n = 2) as well as acquired conditions resulting from chronic endurance exercise (**Fig. 4**).[14]

Noncardiac Diseases

Hyponatremia and exercise-related heatstroke are important causes of noncardiac SD in marathon runners. Hyponatremia in marathon runners potentially leads to cerebral edema, encephalopathy, pulmonary edema, and SD.[19] Although it was shown that approximately 15% of Boston marathon runners in 2002 had asymptomatic hyponatremia, the incidence of potentially serious (symptomatic) hyponatremia is 0.4%.[20] Symptoms include nausea, vomiting, dizziness, headache, and drowsiness. Risk factors include increased fluid intake, female sex, slow finishing times, less marathon exposure, high heat stress weather conditions, and the use of nonsteroidal anti-inflammatory drugs or tricyclic antidepressant drugs.[21–23] Such deaths can be prevented by prerace education on the amount of fluid that should be consumed during the race. Most major

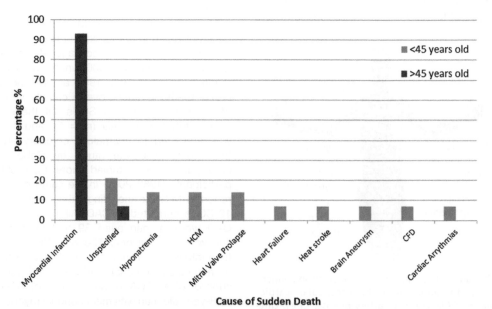

Fig. 4. Causes of sudden death in marathon runners by age group. CFD, coronary fibromuscular dysplasia; HCM, hypertrophic cardiomyopathy. (*Data from* Mathews SC, Narotsky DL, Bernholt DL, et al. Mortality among marathon runners in the United States, 2000–2009. Am J Sports Med 2012;40(7):1495–500.)

marathons ensure that all participants receive advice on their fluid regimen during and after the race, specific for their athletic ability.

Another noncardiac cause of SD in marathon runners is hyperthermia or heatstroke, which accounts for only 3% to 5% of deaths.[14,15] The incidence is 1 in 10,000 marathon finishers and heatstroke is diagnosed when the core temperature is greater than 40°C in the presence of neurologic dysfunction and another sign of organ system failure.[24,25] Risk factors for hyperthermia include racing in hot, humid conditions without adequate hydration, a recent viral illness, and the use of concomitant drugs, such as tricyclic antidepressants and neuroleptic agents that reduce the rate of sweating. Rapid cooling within the first hour ("the golden hour") is the mainstay of therapy.

RISK FACTORS FOR SUDDEN CARDIAC ARREST
Underlying Cardiac Disease

The athletes at greatest risk of SD are those with underlying cardiac disease that may be quiescent and manifest for the first time with SCA during exercise. Most runners (>80%) who have suffered an SCA have not previously reported cardiac symptoms.[12] Although HCM may be compatible with marathon running in some cases,[26] SCA due to HCM in marathon events has a particularly poor prognosis. In addition to the abnormal myocardial substrate, the additional stresses of exercise, notably adrenergic surges and dehydration, are likely to result in diffuse ischemia and dynamic left ventricular obstruction, which likely hinder resuscitation attempts. In contrast, runners with CAD have a considerably better prognosis following SCA with a rate of survival greater than 50%.[15]

Race Distance

Race distance covered has an important impact on rates of SD and planning medical services and placement of automated external defibrillators (AEDs). It has been well documented that the incidence of SCAs in marathons is far greater than that of half marathons, with Kim and colleagues[15] observing incidences of 1.01/100,000 and 0.27/100,000, respectively. The incidence of SD during a marathon increases as the race approaches the finish line (**Fig. 5**). Mathews and colleagues[14] found that the median distance ran before the onset of an SCA was 22.5 miles, with 65% of SCAs (n = 18) occurring at mile 20 or beyond, and 7% within 24 hours of race completion. Kim and colleagues[15] observed that almost 80% of deaths in marathon runners occurred in the last three-quarters of the race.

Sex

Male marathon runners have been shown to be at far greater risk of SCD, with Roberts and colleagues[16] highlighting that over a 30-year period the incidence was 3.8/100,000 and 0.6/100,000 for men and women, respectively. The gender predisposition probably reflects a favorable cardiovascular risk profile of CAD in women as well as a male preponderance of HCM in the general population, which has been quoted as 0.26% in men and 0.09% in women.[27]

PREVENTION OF SUDDEN DEATH
Bystander Cardiopulmonary Resuscitation and Use of Automated External Defibrillators

One of the most fundamental components of an aborted SCA is the rapid initiation of cardiopulmonary resuscitation from a bystander. Such practice increases rates of survival by up to

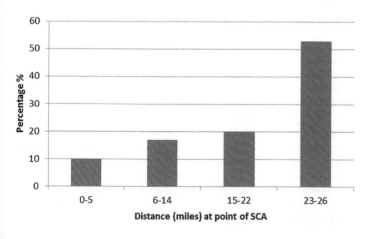

Fig. 5. Relationship between distance run and percentage of SCAs in marathons. SCA, sudden cardiac arrest. (*Data from* Webner D, Duprey KM, Drezner JA, et al. Sudden cardiac arrest and death in United States marathons. Med Sci Sports Exerc 2012; 44(10):1843–5.)

4-fold[15,28] and is integral to the survival of those who suffer an SCA. In the study by Kim and colleagues,[15] bystander cardiopulmonary resuscitation was attempted in 100% of survivors, but only 43% of nonsurvivors. The same study also identified that the time taken for the arrival of emergency medical services as another independent factor to survival. The arrival of emergency medical services was shown to be longer in nonsurvivors than survivors, at a mean of 7.7 and 3.9 minutes, respectively. Rapid use of AEDs in SCA improves survival by several fold and almost certainly explains why rates of resuscitation at sporting events, including survival to discharge range from 16% to 30%, compared with rates of survival in the community, which are in the region of 5%.[29] In the study by Kim and colleagues,[15] 88% of survivors received prompt defibrillation compared with only 35% of nonsurvivors ($P = .03$). It is also time dependent and the highest rates of success are likely if defibrillation is performed within 4 minutes of SCA.[30] AEDs are becoming more commonplace in public areas such as shopping centers and are vital in major event planning, especially sporting events such as the marathon. Their effectiveness stems from their ease of use and widespread availability.

Our understanding of SCD in marathon runners may help major event planning further, and in particular, the placement of AEDs throughout the race course. As stated previously, the risk of SCA correlates with the race distance covered. This correlation is exemplified in a study by Redelmeier and Greenwald,[11] who concluded that the final 1.6 km of the course accounts for less than 5% of the distance but accounts for 50% of sudden cardiac deaths. It is therefore prudent that there is a large concentration of AEDs and cycle responders toward the end stages of the race. Such practice is pertinent considering that rates of survival decrease by 7% to 10% for every minute that defibrillation is delayed.[31]

Preparticipation Screening

Routine cardiac screening in professional competitive sports is now commonplace. However, this is a novel concept in marathons, which attract enormous numbers of participants of varying ages and experience. As CAD is among the commonest causes, some authors have suggested exercise testing as a form of screening.[32] It is well recognized that exercise testing will identify individuals with the most severe disease; however, the inability to detect inducible ischemia in an experienced runner does not exclude a significant

coronary stenosis. Furthermore, it is difficult to simulate marathon running under laboratory conditions and runners with negative exercise tests may still go on to develop demand ischemia and subsequent fatal ventricular arrhythmias during endurance running events.[15,18] It is also important to recognize that routine screening of thousands of marathon participants with exercise testing is not practical or pragmatic. Finally, exercise testing is associated with an unacceptable false positive rate in asymptomatic individuals, particularly women, superseded by newer functional imaging modalities.[33] Most large marathons provide medical information advising only those individuals with symptoms of cardiac disease, a family history of premature cardiac disease, and multiple risk factors for CAD to seek a medical opinion before participation.

Resting electrocardiography testing may identify other causes of SD such as HCM and arrhythmogenic right ventricular cardiomyopathy.[34,35] The yield from such testing can be increased in the presence of prodromal symptoms or a positive family history. The main arguments for routine electrocardiography screening for all marathon runners relate to cost-effectiveness of the strategy as well as issues with false positive tests.[36,37]

Finally, it is important to mention that the number of people dying in marathons is small. A marathon is not a health event; however, it promotes a healthy lifestyle and is likely to reduce the risk of subsequent coronary atheroma in most runners. Although there is a small risk of death in long-distance running, there may actually be a greater risk from other daily activities. A research group in 2007 calculated a 35% relative risk reduction during race time through the prevention of fatal road traffic accidents due to road closures.

REFERENCES

1. Thompson PD, Buchner D, Pina IL, et al. Exercise and physical activity in the prevention and treatment of atherosclerotic cardiovascular disease. Circulation 2003;107(24):3109–16.
2. Agarwal SK. Cardiovascular benefits of exercise. Int J Gen Med 2012;5:541–5.
3. Nelson ME, Rejeski WJ, Blair SN, et al. Physical activity and public health in older adults: recommendation from the American College of Sports Medicine and the American Heart Association. Circulation 2007;116(9):1094–105.
4. Löllgen H, Böckenhoff A, Knapp G. Physical activity and all-cause mortality: an updated meta-analysis with different intensity categories. Int J Sports Med 2009;30(3):213–24.

5. Gremeaux V, Gayda M, Lepers R, et al. Exercise and longevity. Maturitas 2012;73(4):312–7.

6. Chief Medical Officers. Start active, stay active: a report on physical activity for health from the four home countries. London, UK: Department of Health; 2011. Available at: http://www.dh.gov.uk/en/Publicationsandstatistics/Publications/PublicationsPolicyAndGuidance/DH_127931.

7. Haskell WL, Lee IM, Pate RR, et al. Physical activity and public health: updated recommendation for adults from the American College of Sports Medicine and the American Heart Association. Circulation 2007;116(9):1081–93.

8. Wikipedia. Marathon. Available at: http://en.wikipedia.org/wiki/Marathon. Accessed December 20, 2012.

9. Running USA. Running USA Website. Available at: http://www.runningusa.org/. Accessed December 20, 2012.

10. Maron BJ, Poliac LC, Roberts WO. Risk for sudden cardiac death associated with marathon running. J Am Coll Cardiol 1996;29(1):224.

11. Redelmeier DA, Greenwald JA. Competing risks of mortality with marathons: retrospective analysis. BMJ 2007;335(7633):1275–7.

12. Tunstall-Pedoe DS. Marathon cardiac deaths: the London experience. Sports Med 2007;37:448–50.

13. Webner D, Duprey KM, Drezner JA, et al. Sudden cardiac arrest and death in United States marathons. Med Sci Sports Exerc 2012;44(10):1843–5.

14. Mathews SC, Narotsky DL, Bernholt DL, et al. Mortality among marathon runners in the United States, 2000-2009. Am J Sports Med 2012;40(7):1495–500.

15. Kim JH, Malhotra R, Chiampas G, et al. Cardiac arrest during long-distance running races. N Engl J Med 2012;366(2):130–40.

16. Roberts WO, Roberts DM, Lunos S. Marathon related cardiac arrest risk differences in men and women. Br J Sports Med 2012;10(1136):1–4.

17. Cohen SI, Ellis ER. Death and near death from cardiac arrest during the Boston Marathon. Pacing Clin Electrophysiol 2012;35(2):241–4.

18. Sheppard MN. The fittest person in the morgue? Histopathology 2012;60(3):381–96.

19. Goudie AM, Tunstall-Pedoe DS, Kerins M, et al. Exercise-associated hyponatraemia after a marathon: case series. J R Soc Med 2006;99(7):363–7.

20. Almond CS, Shin AY, Fortescue EB, et al. Hyponatremia among runners in the Boston Marathon. N Engl J Med 2005;352(15):1550–6.

21. Hew-butler T, Ayus JC, Kipps C, et al. Statement of the second international exercise-associated hyponatremia consensus development conference, New Zealand, 2007. Clin J Sport Med 2008;18(2):111–21.

22. Rosner MH, Kirven J. Exercise-associated hyponatremia. Clin J Am Soc Nephrol 2007;2(1):151–61.

23. Ayus JC, Varon J, Arieff AI. Hyponatremia, cerebral edema, and noncardiogenic pulmonary edema in marathon runners. Ann Intern Med 2000;132(9):711–4.

24. Roberts WO. Exertional heat stroke in the marathon. Sports Med 2007;37(4–5):440–3.

25. Armstrong LE, Casa DJ, Millard-Stafford M, et al. American College of Sports Medicine position stand. Exertional heat illness during training and competition. Med Sci Sports Exerc 2007;39(3):556–72.

26. Maron BJ, Wesley YE, Arce J. Hypertrophic cardiomyopathy compatible with successful completion of the marathon. Am J Cardiol 1984;53(10):1470–1.

27. Maron BJ, Gardin JM, Flack JM, et al. Prevalence of hypertrophic cardiomyopathy in a general population of young adults. Circulation 1995;92:785–9.

28. Marijon E, Tafflet M, Celermajer DS, et al. Sports-related sudden death in the general population. Circulation 2011;124(6):672–81.

29. Bobrow BJ, Clark LL, Ewy GA, et al. Minimally interrupted cardiac resuscitation by emergency medical services for out-of-hospital cardiac arrest. JAMA 2008;299(10):1158–65.

30. Holmberg M. Factors modifying the effect of bystander cardiopulmonary resuscitation on survival in out-of-hospital cardiac arrest patients in Sweden. Eur Heart J 2001;22(6):511–9.

31. Baum RS, Alvarez H, Cobb LA. Survival after resuscitation from out-of-hospital ventricular fibrillation. Circulation 1974;50(6):1231–5.

32. Day SM, Thompson PD. Cardiac risks associated with marathon running. Sports Health 2010;2(4):301–6.

33. National Institute for Health and Clinical Excellence (NICE). C695 Chest Pain of Recent Onset. London; 2010.

34. Corrado D, Basso C, Pavei A, et al. Trends in sudden cardiovascular death in young competitive athletes. JAMA 2006;296(13):1593–601.

35. Corrado D, Basso C, Schiavon M, et al. Screening for hypertrophic cardiomyopathy in young athletes. N Engl J Med 1998;339(6):364–9.

36. Wheeler MT, Heidenreich PA, Froelicher VF, et al. Cost effectiveness of pre-participation screening for prevention of sudden cardiac death in young athletes. Ann Intern Med 2010;152(5):276–86.

37. Maron BJ, Thompson PD, Ackerman MJ, et al. Recommendations and considerations related to preparticipation screening for cardiovascular abnormalities in competitive athletes. Circulation 2007;115(12):1643–55.

Exercise Testing for Risk Stratification of Ventricular Arrhythmias in the Athlete

Christian Schmied, MD*, Corinna Brunckhorst, MD,
Firat Duru, MD, Laurent Haegeli, MD

KEYWORDS

- Exercise testing • Exercise-induced ventricular arrhythmia (EIVA)
- Premature ventricular beats (PVBs) • Catecholaminergic polymorphic ventricular tachycardia (CPVT)

KEY POINTS

- Exercise testing is an important diagnostic tool that creates an environment of automaticity at the electrical membrane, which tolerates premature beats and re-entrant arrhythmogenic circuits.
- Exercise testing mimics the authentic situation of physical activity and stress, which has been recognized as a fatal trigger of critical arrhythmias in cases of underlying cardiac risk constellation.
- Although it is established as a second-line diagnostic tool, exercise testing can provide crucial information in an earlier setting, if
  - exercise-dependent symptoms in an athlete's history (eg, tachyarrhythmia, lightheadedness, and fainting/syncope) are present.
  - there is clinical suspicion of an underlying structural or primarily electrical heart disease that can be further evaluated by the use of an exercise test.
  - there is known structural or electrical disease for which exercise testing provides crucial information concerning management and prognosis of the disease.

INTRODUCTION AND PHYSIOLOGIC ADAPTATIONS DURING EXERCISE

Generally, the classic baseline cardiac screening in young athletes consists of a focused physical examination, a standardized questionnaire, and, most importantly, a 12-lead resting ECG.[1] As Italian data impressively demonstrated, the addition of a 12-lead resting ECG proved to be the crux of the matter, leading to dramatic reductions of incidences of fatal cardiac events in sports.[2–4] Although a resting ECG reliably detects underlying structural or electrical cardiac disease, it does not reproduce the authentic situation of physical activity and stress, which is recognized as a fatal trigger of critical arrhythmias in cases of an underlying cardiac risk constellation.[5–9] Due to the potential of many false-positive findings and the lack of cost effectiveness, standardized exercise testing is usually not integrated in the baseline screening of young athletes under the age of 35.[1,10,11] It is a crucial issue in the evaluation of older athletes, in which coronary heart disease (CHD), in particular, myocardial infarction (MI), is by far the most common cause of sudden cardiac death (SCD) in sports.[11,12] Particularly if athletes older than 35 show an elevated risk for CHD with the potential for exercise-induced MI, consensus panels recommend the addition of an exercise test.[11,13] In addition to the interpretation of ST segments, however, to unmask exercise-induced MI, exercise testing provides information referring to physical capacity as well as blood pressure and heart rate adaptations during exercise.

Disclosures: No conflicts of interest to declare.
Cardiovascular Centre, Division of Cardiology, University Hospital Zürich, Raemistrasse 100, Zürich 8091, Switzerland
* Corresponding author. Clinic for Cardiology, Cardiovascular Center, Division of Cardiology, University Hospital Zürich, Raemistrasse 100, Zürich 8091, Switzerland.
E-mail address: christian.schmied@usz.ch

Card Electrophysiol Clin 5 (2013) 53–64
http://dx.doi.org/10.1016/j.ccep.2012.11.003
1877-9182/13/$ – see front matter © 2013 Elsevier Inc. All rights reserved.

Last but not least, exercise testing can be an important tool to detect, categorize, and follow-up various arrhythmias.[14] Finally, it may be of prognostic value: some studies documented a 12-month mortality that is 3 times greater in persons exhibiting exercise-induced ectopy than those with ectopy at rest only,[15] and in patients with exercise-induced arrhythmia, mortality of those with complex ectopy exceeds that of those with simple ectopy.[16]

The classic example of a highly malignant, primarily electric condition, in the absence of an underlying structural disease, which can be reproduced during exercise, is catecholaminergic polymorphic ventricular tachycardia (CPVT), in particular, familial polymorphic ventricular tachycardia. A detailed overview of this disease is discussed later.

Nevertheless, exercise testing is able to provide important information regarding malignancy and prognosis of other primarily electrical or structural cardiopathies, such as long QT syndrome (LQTS), hypertrophic cardiomyopathy (HCM), Chagas disease, CHD, and so forth. In cases of mandatory medical treatment, exercise testing can be crucial in the evaluation of therapy success and drug dose regimen (eg, β-blockers and type Ic antiarrhythmics). Finally the clinical significance of premature ventricular beats (PVBs), in particular, unspecific exercise-induced ventricular arrhythmias (EIVAs) in eventually normal hearts whose clinical implications are less clear is also discussed.[17] Although some investigators suggest the extrapolation of the number of PVBs assessed by resting ECG, the dynamic characteristics of the PVBs under conditions of physical exercise have proved crucial.[18,19]

Physiologic Adaptations and Mechanisms During Exercise

What are the underlying physiologic adaptations that lead to specific conditions triggering ventricular arrhythmia during exercise? The activated sympathetic nervous system increases circulating catecholamines, which can create an environment of automaticity at the electrical membrane that tolerates premature beats and re-entrant arrhythmogenic circuits.[18] Whether the electrical mechanism consists of re-entry mechanism, enhanced automaticity, or after-depolarizations is a matter of debate.[19] Irrespective of these questions, exercise-induced variations of electrical patterns (eg, short-long-short RR interval sequence or a regular RR pattern) may provoke EIVAs.[18]

Additionally, ventricular arrhythmias can be triggered by electrolyte imbalance, transient ischemia, myocardial stretch, and/or activation.[19]

At the cellular base, sympathoadrenergic tone leads to $Ca2+$-induced $Ca2+$ release by protein kinase A–mediated phosphorylation of type 2 ryanodine receptors (RyR2)—the crucial mechanism underlying cardiac excitation–contraction coupling.[20] Calcium influx into the cardiomyocytes through the sarcolemmal L-type calcium channels is followed by $Ca2+$-induced release of additional $Ca2+$ ions from the lumen of the sarcoplasmic reticulum into the cytosol via RyR2.[20]

The role of potassium concentrations, in particular, during vigorous exertion was discussed in former studies: although alterations of potassium levels may facilitate ventricular arrhythmia, generally they seem well tolerated. Even more than that: although vigorous exercise may lead to a doubling of serum potassium concentration (with concomitant decrease of pH-values) and a 10-fold increase of catecholamine levels, an interaction between these mechanisms may even lead to a protecting effect from stress-induced chemical damage (calcium currents inwards may stabilize the integrity of potassium-depolarized action potential at the myocyte).[21] These protecting mechanisms are diminished not only in the setting of myocardial ischemia but also physiologically during recovery when plasma potassium is low, although adrenergic tone remains high. That is one major argument for the strict necessity of an adequate cool-down protocol.[18,21]

Pathophysiologic Changes During Exercise Triggering Ventricular Arrhythmias

The relationship between vigorous physical exercise and transient increase in the risk of sudden death due to ventricular arrhythmias was first recognized decades ago.[6,22] This holds true particularly for men with no or low levels of habitual activity.[7] Because the majority of sudden deaths only occurs in subjects with an underlying organic or primarily electrical cardiac pathology, physical exercise is believed to further precipitate the initiation of ventricular arrhythmias and/or maintain these events in an already arrhythmogenic substrate. From an electrophysiologic perspective, ventricular arrhythmias occur as a result of complex interaction of factors, such as arrhythmogenic substrate (underlying cardiac pathology), triggering events (PVBs), and regulators (ischemia, electrolyte disturbances, hemodynamic and autonomic disturbances, and so forth). A marked increase in sympathetic activity due to excessive physical effort and associated emotional stress not only increases the occurrence of extrasystoles as triggers of ventricular arrhythmias but also promotes abrupt increase of myocardial oxygen demand. In patients with CHD, the latter condition may lead to plaque rupture with subsequent thrombus formation, which may be manifested as acute coronary events with resultant ventricular arrhythmias, especially in individuals who did not have regular exercise habits. This is in contrast to individuals who exercise regularly in whom the overall risk of coronary events is less due to prevention of development or progression of CHD. Likewise, myocardial ischemia may be a precipitator of ventricular arrhythmias in young athletes with coronary artery anomalies.

The pathophysiology of arrhythmic events in individuals who perform excessive endurance exercise has been a matter of debate. Complex ventricular ectopy, ventricular tachyarrhythmias, and SCD can even occur in fit athletes.[23] Autonomic nervous system adaptations induced by endurance training have been reported to have a role in the genesis of ventricular tachyarrhythmias in subjects who are susceptible to occurrence of these events.[24–26] It is likely that a shift in autonomic modulation from parasympathetic to sympathetic predominance due to intensive training regimen may predispose the athletes to electrical instability, triggering ventricular tachyarrhythmias.[27]

Pathologic underlying conditions may enhance and accelerate physiologic sequences. These preconditions may affect relevant conduction channels (calcium, sodium, and potassium), structural microanatomic or macroanatomic cardiac changes, pharmacologic influences (eg, proarrhythmogenic drugs), or the response to exercise itself. In this context, some studies suggest that inherited structural cardiopathies may not solely explain the underlying condition—regular exercise itself may lead to transient structural adaptations (eg, of the right ventricle) that vice versa may lead to a proarrhythmogenic state.[28] There is evidence supporting the hypothesis that in some subjects who perform long-term strenuous endurance efforts, such as marathon running or cycling, cardiac fibrosis may occur, especially in the right ventricle, the interventricular septum, and the atria, resulting in increased susceptibility to ventricular and atrial arrhythmias.[29] There is also accumulating evidence suggesting the occurrence of adverse structural remodeling, which is most apparent in right-sided cardiac chambers.[30–32] Hormonal alterations, such as changes in plasma cortisol levels induced by prolonged and intensive training, may have possible influence on myocardial irritability, triggering ventricular tachyarrhythmias.[33] Last but not least, there is also biomarker evidence for cardiac damage with extreme endurance training, which may cause a direct toxic effect triggering arrhythmic events.[34,35] Nevertheless, the true clinical significance of elevated cardiac biomarkers after exercise remains uncertain because this is usually a transient event.

EXERCISE TESTING IN ATHLETES WITH KNOWN CARDIOVASCULAR DISEASE

Although frequently thorough restrictions are mandatory—based on currently well-established expert panel consensus statements,[36,37] competitive sport based on specially tailored protocols is possible and requested in most cases of underlying cardiovascular disease.

In this setting, exercise tests have an important role not only in the assessment of CHD: In particular, the estimation of exercise-induced myocardial ischemia, but also of exercise-related blood pressure, heart rate, and heart rhythm behavior indicates information concerning eligibility for competitive sports and effectiveness of medical treatment.[36,37]

Exercise Testing in Athletes with Underlying Structural Disease

The underlying structural diseases discussed in this section include

- HCM
- Arrhythmogenic right ventricular cardiomyopathy (ARVC)
- Chagas disease
- Congenital heart disease

Hypertrophic cardiomyopathy

The pathophysiology of ventricular tachyarrhythmias in HCM involves a complex arrhythmogenic substrate formed by disarray of myocardial cells along with fibrosis and calcium regulation abnormalities, which predisposes the subject to occurrence of life-threatening events. Although patients with known HCM are usually restricted from any competitive sports, the impact of exercise testing and arrhythmia during exercise can be exemplarily demonstrated. Numerous studies have shown that the presence of nonsustained ventricular tachycardia (NSVT) during ambulatory Holter monitoring is associated with an estimated 2-fold to 2.5-fold increase in sudden death risk, particularly in young adults and children with the disease.[38–42] In one study, a midmorning peak of NSVT was observed.[43] Although the biologic basis for the circadian pattern is debatable, the timing suggests an influence of vagal tone.[39–41] Only few studies, however, reported on ventricular tachycardia (VT) during exercise. Although one study was unable to determine its prognostic significance,[44] a recent survey recognized an increased risk of SCD associated with frequent ventricular arrhythmia during exercise in HCM patients.[45] These findings emphasize the importance of exercise testing in the risk stratification in patients with HCM and suggest that exercise-induced NSVT should be taken into account, besides other factors, when assessing the need for an implantable cardioverter-defibrillator.

Arrhythmogenic right ventricular cardiomyopathy

Patients with ARVC are particularly vulnerable to arrhythmic events because the disease-specific myocardial atrophy and fibrofatty infiltration leads to a very arrhythmogenic underlying substrate. Although the prognostic impact has not been proved, exercise testing is routinely included in the diagnostic evaluation of patients with suspected ARVC.[46–51] A recent review concluded that the response of ventricular ectopic activity to exercise is highly variable in young patients with ARVC, and the diagnostic utility of graded exercise testing is thus questionable in young patients with suspected ARVC.[52] The absence or suppression of VPCs during exercise should not be considered reassuring in terms of diagnostic exclusion of disease.[50]

Chagas disease

Although not (yet?) a major issue in Europe, Chagas disease is a major medical and social problem throughout most of Latin America and cardiac affection is frequent.[53–55] Chagas heart disease can be seen as an arrhythmic cardiomyopathy, and frequent, complex PVBs, including runs of VT, are a common finding.[56,57] In particular, EIVAs suggest an independent prognostic risk factor of the disease, particularly in association with other factors, such as cardiomegaly on radiograph or low left ventricular ejection fraction.

Congenital heart disease

As with most cardiovascular diseases, in athletes with congenital heart disease, the benefit of sports on physical and mental health outweighs its potential harm. Only patients with congenital heart disease who are likely to deteriorate and are at high risk of life-threatening arrhythmias should be restricted from sports participation. It is a hallmark of congenital heart disease that, compared with individuals assumed stable at rest, relevant hemodynamic changes are demonstrated during exercise. The assessment of arrhythmia during exercise deserves a special focus in these athletes.[36,37] Particularly widened QRS complexes (duration >160 ms) can be interpreted as a warning sign for the susceptibility to proarrhythmic situations.[36,37]

In athletes with known congenital heart disease, exercise testing is a cornerstone of medical assessment, particularly by analyzing ST segment changes during exercise to detect exercise-induced myocardial ischemia. Recent trials, furthermore, have shown a poor long-term follow-up prognosis in concomitant congenital heart disease and EIVAs.[19,58] In large samples of patients with known CHD, EIVAs during recovery are a strong predictor of death.[59]

Exercise Testing in Athletes with Underlying Electrical Disease

Long QT syndrome

LQTS, first described in 1957,[60] is characterized by an abnormal and prolonged repolarization, either congenital or acquired. Overall, LQTS is a rare condition with an estimated prevalence of 0.4% in athletes.[61] The prevalence of LQTS is difficult to estimate, however. Given the currently increasing frequency of diagnoses, LQTS may be expected to occur in 1 in 10,000 individuals. But it remains an underdiagnosed disorder, especially because at least 10% to 15% of LQTS gene carriers have a normal QTc duration.

So far, 12 different types of LQTS have been described, of which LQTS 1–3 play the most important role clinically. Generally, in LQTS1, SCD is associated with physical exertion; in LQTS2, it is linked to autonomic nervous arousal and stress and in LQTS 3 with increased vagal tone at rest and with bradycardia.[62] Although critical QTc cutoffs are widely accepted (0.47 seconds and 0.48 seconds for male and female athletes, respectively[63]), definite diagnosis remains challenging in up to 50% of patients with LQTS that can show a normal to borderline prolonged QT interval (concealed LQTS).[64–66] As a gold standard, genetic testing remains expensive and unavailable to many centers, although it is a reliable tool to identify phenotypic-negative patients with LQTS. Furthermore, genetic testing may identify novel LQTS mutations of undefined significance (eg, false-positive, single-nucleotide polymorphisms).[67] Exercise testing represents a reasonable strategy not only to provoke and unmask the LQTS phenotype but also to validate significance of unspecific genetic findings. In a recent study, Wong and colleagues[68] confirmed former findings and demonstrated that (concealed) LQTS patients had a greater prolongation of their QTc interval with changes in posture than controls. It is well-known that failed QT shortening, in particular, QT prolongation during exercise, is highly suggestive of LQT1, because the LQT1 gene encodes for the IKs potassium channel, which is responsible for the repolarization phase of the cardiac cycle at rapid heart rates.[68]

In a landmark study of Takenaka and colleagues,[69] exercise testing in combination with qualitative assessment of T-wave morphology was useful in identifying patients with LQT1 mutations. The identification of LQT2 patients, however, was more limited in this study because it was dependent on the qualitative assessment of T-wave morphology changes during exercise. As Wong and colleagues[68] demonstrated, patients with LQT1 mutations also showed a well-expected and marked QTc prolongation during exercise, whereas LQT2 patients had an exaggerated QT hysteresis compared with LQT1 and controls. Larger studies are needed, however, to confirm these findings.

Wolff-Parkinson-White syndrome

Individuals with Wolff-Parkinson-White (WPW) syndrome, in particular those having accessory pathways with short refractory periods, are at risk for ventricular fibrillation (VF) due to rapid atrioventricular conduction during atrial fibrillation.[70] Therefore, risk stratification in athletes with WPW syndrome is important given the small risk of SCD.[70] Nevertheless, SCD may be the first presentation of the syndrome in up to 1.4% of patients.[71] Because most guidelines do not recommend routine invasive electrophysiologic assessment in asymptomatic patients, other noninvasive methods for risk stratifying asymptomatic patients with ventricular pre-excitation have been evaluated. Intermittent loss of pre-excitation due to increased heart rate during exercise testing previously has been shown to have a high negative predictive value for SCD due to the presumed inability of the accessory pathway to conduct rapidly at higher atrial rates.[72] Nevertheless, some experts have recommended invasive electrophysiologic assessment in all patients with WPW, regardless of symptoms, and this seems reasonable particularly for competitive athletes.[36,37,71]

Exercise Testing in Athletes on Antiarrhythmic Drug Therapy

In patients on antiarrhythmic therapy, sustained exercise-induced VT is associated with a high risk of sudden death.[16]

Type IC drugs are a reasonable and well-established therapy to maintain sinus rhythm in athletes with lone atrial fibrillation.[73] Due to proarrhythmic effects, however, all antiarrhythmic drugs used to maintain sinus rhythm have the potential to increase ectopy or induce or aggravate monomorphic ventricular tachycardia (VT), torsades de pointes, or VF. In type Ic antiarrhythmics, QRS widening should not be permitted to exceed 120% to 130% of the baseline QRS duration, and exercise testing is classically the method of choice to detect QRS widening that occurs only at rapid heart rates (use-dependent conduction slowing). In this setting, exercise testing is also useful to screen for exercise-induced arrhythmia and is typically performed 1 to 2 weeks after drug initiation or dose increase.[73]

CLINICAL SIGNIFICANCE OF EXERCISE-INDUCED VENTRICULAR ARRHYTHMIAS

PVBs are a common finding in athletes although they seem to occur with the same frequency as they do in the general population.[19,74] The disappearance of PVBs with exercise is the normal case and implicates a favorable prognosis.[19,75] Despite that, they sometimes provoke anxiety in athletes—and their doctors.

Clinical and prognostic implications are not entirely explained[19] and although many studies found a favorable prognosis[76–78] of increased PVBs at rest—particularly in athletes—some groups postulate a certain burden of PVBs in athletes as a strong predictor of adverse cardiac risk.[79–84] The number of PVBs can either be estimated on the base of a resting ECG or assessed by 24-hour Holter monitoring.[19,85,86] Biffi and colleagues[85,86] studied the prognostic impact of ventricular arrhythmia in 24-hour Holter monitoring in competitive athletes: ventricular arrhythmia proved common; nevertheless, this finding was usually not associated with underlying cardiovascular abnormalities.

Generally, the prevalence of EIVA increases in older populations[87–89] and in those with CV disease[87,90,91]; thus, it could be supposed that EIVAs may result from exercise-induced ischemia.[88,91,92] Nevertheless, in large samples of patients with known CHD[59] and also in athletes,[19,75] EIVAs during recovery are a strong predictor of a serious prognosis.

Data on the implications of exercise-induced PVBs are inconclusive, however.[17,87,93] The majority of the studies focused on the predictive value of exercise-induced PVBs in patients referred for diagnostic exercise testing.[15,59,88,94,95] Nevertheless, although most surveys[15,88,89,95,96] showed no correlation between exercise-induced PVBs and all-cause mortality, others suggest that EIVAs may indicate a poor prognosis.[15,88,94,97] A recent study found that healthy volunteers with EIVAs proved to have increased mortality.[91,98] Another large study determined that frequent PVBs occurring after exercise might be more predictive of mortality than PVBs occurring during exercise.[19]

It is delicate, however, to compare most of the surveys due to their significant differences in study design and protocols. Exemplary mismatches consist of some studies isolating hard cardiovascular endpoints from secondary cardiovascular endpoints. Furthermore, some investigators defined frequent PVBs differently from other studies, whereas some investigators separated the entity of EIVAs from PVBs at rest completely and excluded individuals with PVBs at rest.[75]

An adequate comparison is also not admissible if exercise and ECG monitoring protocols as well as follow-up strategies differed. In addition, the age groups and inclusion of women varied between the studies, and there were probably differences in racial diversity and cardiovascular risk behavior.

So, how can a rational conclusion be reached? It seems reasonable to assume that the presence of PVBs, per se, implicates an environment of increased electrical excitability and that their association with exercise suggests catecholamine sensitivity.

At the bottom line, most of the studies suggest that EIVAs do not clearly predict an increased cardiovascular risk in normal hearts, at least over the short time. Nevertheless, athletes should be monitored by regular cardiac assessments, including careful history, physical examination, resting ECG, and probably echocardiogram. Repetitive exercise tests and probably Holter monitoring can detect progression to high-grade arrhythmia, particularly in the case of symptoms.

Finally, the hypothesis that exercise-induced PVB may identify patients at risk for noncardiovascular deaths warrants additional large cohort studies. Additionally, the relation between EIVAs and cardiovascular endpoints should be focused in further investigations.

A minor observation is that a strict distinction between ventricular arrhythmia at rest and during exercise is not advisable in any case: Froelicher and Lemberg[18] demonstrated that individuals with both resting PVB and EIVAs seem at highest risk for adverse cardiac events. Additionally, exercise-induced supraventricular arrhythmias may increase the risk of developing atrial fibrillation.

CATECHOLAMINERGIC POLYMORPHIC VENTRICULAR TACHYCARDIA—THE CLASSICAL EXERCISE-DEPENDENT ENTITY

Beside some other syndromes, such as right ventricular outflow tract tachycardia in a normal heart, where VT may be reproducibly induced during exercise testing, CPVT is the classical exercise-dependent entity—first described in the 1970s.[99] Patients at a young age with structurally normal hearts and normal 12-lead ECGs present with bidirectional or polymorphic VT, which are repeatedly induced by conditions of increased sympathetic activity, like physical exercise or acute

emotional stress. This arrhythmic condition manifests mostly as syncope or cardiac arrest if VT degenerates into VF.[100] Specific gene mutations encoding proteins responsible for calcium release from the sarcoplasmic reticulum result in abnormal calcium handling in cardiac cells. The resulting cytosolic calcium overload leads to delayed afterdepolarizations, triggered activity, and ventricular arrhythmias, especially under conditions of enhanced β-adrenergic tone. In 60% of patients with CPVT, mutations encoding for cardiac RYR2 or less frequently for cardiac calsequestrin 2 are identified, which are associated with autosomal dominant and recessive transmission, respectively.[101,102]

Untreated patients with CPVT have a 79% incidence of cardiac events up to 40 years of age. The incidence of SCD is 30%.[103] Since the detection of the strong relationship between VT and β-adrenergic activation in patients with CPVT, the efficacy of β-blocker therapy was recognized and established as a cornerstone in the treatment of CPVT patients. β-blockers are the most effective drugs to reduce ventricular arrhythmias during exercise testing or Holter monitoring and to prevent arrhythmic events.[100]

Despite efficient protection in a majority of patients by β-blocker therapy, arrhythmic events are observed in up to one-third of the patients. In these cases, the implantation of a defibrillator may be warranted. In the current American College of Cardiology (ACC)/American Heart Association (AHA)/European Society of Cardiology guidelines for management of patients with ventricular arrhythmias and the prevention of SCD, the implantation of a defibrillator is considered a class 1 recommendation for CPVT patients who survived a cardiac arrest. Although defibrillators have been implanted by cardiologists liberally, defibrillator therapy may have malignant proarrhythmic effects in CPVT patients because both appropriate and inappropriate shocks can trigger catecholamine release, leading to subsequent electrical storm, multiple shocks, and death.

Flecainide drug therapy could be considered an adjunctive treatment in cases of recurrent arrhythmias despite β-blocker therapy because studies in a CPVT mouse model suggest that flecainide was able to suppress arrhythmia.[104]

In the acute treatment of ventricular storm or VF in CPVT patients, standard intravenous epinephrine therapy in a resuscitation setting should be avoided and β-blocker therapy given as a first choice. General anesthesia would be the last option if β-blocker therapy fails.

Genetic screening for family members to identify silent mutation carriers with no ventricular arrhythmias inducible by exercise testing is important because these patients have an increased risk for arrhythmic events, which can be reduced by antiadrenergic therapy.[105] Furthermore, advising against participation in competitive sports and prohibiting the use of sympathomimetic agents is important.

EXERCISE TESTING IN CARDIAC SCREENING OF COMPETITIVE ATHLETES

As discussed in this article, exercise testing provides a wealth of crucial information. This diagnostic tool needs to be applied, however, only in specific situations. It may not be surprising that exercise testing is not recommended as a first-line tool in cardiac screening of competitive athletes,[1,4] whether young or older athletes, where it eventually provides crucial information concerning exercise-induced myocardial ischemia. Only in cases of at least moderately increased risk for atherosclerosis and CHD in athletes older than 30 to 35 years undergoing routine stress testing is recommended.[11] In a recent publication, Sofi and collaborators[106] studied 30,065 athletes who underwent an exercise test before participation in competitive sports. They found that age greater than 30 years was significantly associated with an increased risk of being disqualified for cardiac findings during exercise testing.

Exercise testing, however, reproduces a realistic condition of physical activity and resembles a situation an athlete is frequently exposed to and during which symptoms are probably experienced. It is a valuable and feasible diagnostic tool in the evaluation of athletes, constituting an alternative to ambulatory ECG monitoring.

In adrenergic-dependent rhythm disturbances (including monomorphic VT as well as polymorphic VT related to LQTSs), ambulatory ECG monitoring may fail to supply the circumstances necessary for induction of VT, particularly if a patient is sedentary and the arrhythmia is infrequent.[17,107]

Apart from older athletes, in whom accurate cardiovascular risk assessment should precede exercise testing due to the high rate of potentially false-positive findings, the main indications for exercise testing are as follows:

- Exercise-dependent symptoms in an athlete's history (eg, tachyarrhythmia, light-headedness, or fainting/syncope)
- Clinical suspicion of an underlying structural or primarily electrical heart disease that can be further evaluated by the use of an exercise test

- Known structural or electrical disease in which exercise testing provides crucial information concerning management and prognosis of the disease

The 1997 ACC and the AHA recommendations for exercise testing were updated in 2002 (**Table 1**).[17,107] For the "investigation of heart rhythm disorders" a class I recommendation has only been declared for the identification of an appropriate setting in patients with rate-adaptive pacemakers and the evaluation of congenital complete heart block in patients considering increased physical activity or participation in competitive sports (level of evidence: C). The evaluation of patients with known or suspected exercise-induced arrhythmias received a class IIa recommendation and is indicated if the baseline assessment (mainly athletes' personal and family history and ECG) suggests an underlying exercise-related cardiopathy. Furthermore, athletes with exercise-related symptoms (eg, syncope) should also undergo a stress test, according to these nonathlete-specific recommendations. Although the investigation of isolated ventricular ectopic beats by an exercise test is only recommended in middle-aged patients without other evidence of CHD (class IIb), it is not recommended in nonathletic young patients (class III recommendation). The investigation of prolonged first-degree atrioventricular block or type I second-degree Wenckebach, left bundle-branch block, right bundle-branch block, or isolated ectopic beats in young patients considering participation in competitive sports received a class IIb recommendation as well (level of evidence: C).

In cases of exercise-associated symptoms, the exercise test should be performed in a sports-related manner, whenever possible (eg, runners and football players on a treadmill or cyclists on a bike). Apart from individual sports, however, some specific features should be respected: both treadmill and cycle ergometer devices are commonly used, but although cycle ergometers are generally less expensive, smaller, and less noisy than treadmills and produce less motion of the upper body, the fatigue of the quadriceps muscles in patients who are not experienced cyclists is a major limitation, because subjects usually stop before reaching their maximum oxygen uptake. As a result, treadmills are more commonly used in the United States.[17,107] In screening for exercise-related arrhythmia, however, the authors usually prefer the cycle ergometer because ECG artifacts are less frequent.

Furthermore, it should be emphasized that the choice of exercise protocol may influence cardiovascular (and arrhythmic) response. Various

Table 1
Investigation of heart rhythm disorders (ACC/AHA recommendations for exercise testing; update 2002)

Class I	Class IIa	Class III
1. Identification of appropriate settings in patients with rate-adaptive pacemakers 2. Evaluation of congenital complete heart block in patients considering increased physical activity or participation in competitive sports (level of evidence: C)	1. Evaluation of patients with known or suspected exercise-induced arrhythmias 2. Evaluation of medical, surgical, or ablative therapy in patients with exercise-induced arrhythmias (including atrial fibrillation) **Class IIb** 1. Investigation of isolated ventricular ectopic beats in middle-aged patients without other evidence of CHD 2. Investigation of prolonged first-degree atrioventricular block or type I second degree Wenckebach, left bundle-branch block, right bundle-branch block, or isolated ectopic beats in young patients considering participation in competitive sports (level of evidence: C)	1. Routine investigation of isolated ectopic beats in young patients

From Gibbons RJ, Balady GJ, Bricker JT, et al. ACC/AHA 2002 guideline update for exercise testing: summary article: a report of the American College of Cardiology/American Heart Association Task Force on Practice Guidelines (Committee to Update the 1997 Exercise Testing Guidelines). Circulation 2002;106:1883–92; with permission.

protocols have been assessed to find an optimal way to provoke and unmask underlying cardiopathies and arrhythmia. Although much of the published data are based on the Bruce protocol, there are advantages to customizing the protocol to individual athletes to allow 8 to 12 minutes of exercise.[108] Although ramp protocols have been widely accepted as the optimal protocol to detect exercise-induced myocardial ischemia, no specific protocols have been found to provoke arrhythmias in particular (eg, the so-called 4-second exercise test).[109]

Finally, it must be emphasized that even in a population with suspected serious exercise-induced arrhythmia, testing can be performed with low mortality and few lasting morbid events.[110]

REFERENCES

1. Corrado D, Pelliccia A, Bjørnstad HH, et al. Cardiovascular preparticipation screening of young competitive athletes for prevention of sudden death: proposal for a common European protocol: consensus statement of the Study Group of Sport Cardiology of the Working Group of Cardiac Rehabilitation and Exercise Physiology and the Working Group of Myocardial and Pericardial Diseases of the European Society of Cardiology. Eur Heart J 2005;26:516–20.
2. Corrado D, Basso C, Thiene G. Assay: sudden death in young athletes. Lancet 2005;45:47–8.
3. Corrado D, Basso C, Pavei A, et al. Trends in sudden cardiovascular death in young competitive athletes after implementation of a preparticipation screening program. JAMA 2006;296:1593–601.
4. Maron BJ, Haas TS, Doerer JJ, et al. Comparison of U.S. and Italian experiences with sudden cardiac deaths in young competitive athletes and implications for preparticipation screening strategies. Am J Cardiol 2009;104:276–80.
5. Maron BJ. The paradox of exercise. N Engl J Med 2000;343:1409–11.
6. Thompson PD, Funk EJ, Carleton RA, et al. Incidence of death during jogging in Rhode Island from 1975 through 1980. JAMA 1982;247:2535–8.
7. Siscovick DS, Weiss NS, Fletcher RH, et al. The incidence of primary cardiac arrest during vigorous exercise. N Engl J Med 1984;311:874–7.
8. Corrado D, Thiene G, Nava A, et al. Sudden death in young competitive athletes: clinico-pathologic correlations in 22 cases. Am J Med 1990;89:588–96.

9. Maron BJ. Sudden death in young athletes. N Engl J Med 2003;349:1064–75.

10. Maron BJ, Thompson PD, Ackerman MJ, et al. Recommendations and considerations related to preparticipation screening for cardiovascular abnormalities in competitive athletes: 2007 update: a scientific statement from the American Heart Association Council on Nutrition, Physical Activity, and Metabolism: endorsed by the American College of Cardiology Foundation. Circulation 2007;115:1643–55.

11. Corrado D, Schmied C, Basso C, et al. Risk of sports: do we need a pre-participation screening for competitive and leisure athletes? Eur Heart J 2011;32(8):934–44.

12. Corrado D, Migliore F, Basso C, et al. Exercise and the risk of sudden cardiac death. Herz 2006;31:553–8.

13. Rodgers GP, Ayanian JZ, Balady G, et al. American College of Cardiology/American Heart Association Clinical Competence Statement on Stress Testing. A Report of the American College of Cardiology/ American Heart Association/American College of Physicians-American Society of Internal Medicine Task Force on Clinical Competence. Circulation 2000;102:1726–38.

14. Woelfel A, Foster JR, Simpson RJ, et al. Reproducibility and treatment of exercise-induced ventricular tachycardia. Am J Cardiol 1984;53:751–6.

15. Califf RM, McKinnis RA, McNeer JF, et al. Prognostic value of ventricular arrhythmias associated with treadmill exercise testing in patients studied with cardiac catheterization for suspected ischemic heart disease. J Am Coll Cardiol 1983;2(6):1060–7.

16. Graboys TB, Lown B, Podrid PJ, et al. Long-term survival of patients with malignant ventricular arrhythmia treated with antiarrhythmic drugs. Am J Cardiol 1982;50(3):437–43.

17. Gibbons RJ, Balady GJ, Beasley JW, et al. ACC/ AHA guidelines for exercise testing: a report of the American College of Cardiology/American Heart Association Task force on practice guidelines. J Am Coll Cardiol 1997;30:260–311 [updated Circulation. 2002;106(14):1883–92].

18. Futterman LG, Lemberg L. The clinical significance of exercise-induced ventricular arrhythmias. Am J Crit Care 2006;15:431–5.

19. Selzman KA, Gettes LS. Exercise-induced premature ventricular beats: should we do anything differently? Circulation 2004;109:2374–5.

20. Kontula K, Laitinen PJ, Lehtonen A, et al. Catecholaminergic polymorphic ventricular tachycardia: recent mechanistic insights. Cardiovasc Res 2005;67:379–87.

21. Beckerman J, Wu T, Jones S, et al. Exercise testinduced arrhythmias. Prog Cardiovasc Dis 2005;47:285–305.

22. Paffenbarger RS Jr, Wing AL, Hyde RT. Physical activity as an index of heart attack risk in college alumni. Am J Epidemiol 1978;108(3):161–75.

23. Kim JH, Malhotra R, Chiampas G, et al. Cardiac arrest during long-distance running races. N Engl J Med 2012;366(2):130–40.

24. Fazio G, Novo G, Sutera L, et al. Sympathetic tone and ventricular tachycardia. J Cardiovasc Med 2008;9:963–6.

25. Chen LS, Zhou S, Fishbein MC, et al. New perspectives on the role of autonomic nervous system in the genesis of arrhythmias. J Cardiovasc Electrophysiol 2007;18:123–7.

26. Ueno LM, Moritani T. Effects of long-term exercise training on cardiac autonomic nervous activities and baroreflex sensitivity. Eur J Appl Physiol 2003;89:109–14.

27. Iellamo F, Legramante JM, Pigozzi F, et al. Conversion from vagal to sympathetic predominance with strenuous training in high-performance world class athletes. Circulation 2002;105:2719–24.

28. Heidbuchel H, Hoogsteen J, Fagard R, et al. High prevalence of right ventricularinvolvement in endurance athletes with ventricular arrhythmias. Role of an electrophysiologic study in risk stratification. Eur Heart J 2003;24:1473–80.

29. O'Keefe JH, Patil HR, Lavie CJ, et al. Potential adverse cardiovascular effects from excessive endurance exercise. Mayo Clin Proc 2012;87(6):587–95.

30. Nassenstein K, Breuckmann F, Lehmann N, et al. Left ventricular volumes and mass in marathon runners and their association with cardiovascular risk factors. Int J Cardiovasc Imaging 2009;25(1):71–9.

31. Ector J, Ganame J, van der Merwe N, et al. Reduced right ventricular ejection fraction in endurance athletes presenting with ventricular arrhythmias: a quantitative angiographic assessment. Eur Heart J 2007;28(3):345–53.

32. Maron BJ, Pelliccia A. The heart of trained athletes: cardiac remodeling and the risks of sports, including sudden death. Circulation 2006;114(15):1633–44.

33. Bonifazi M, Sardella F, Lupo C. Preparatory versus main competitions: differences in performances, lactate responses and pre-competition plasma cortisol concentrations in elite male swimmers. Eur J Appl Physiol 2000;82:368–73.

34. Neilan TG, Januzzi JL, Lee-Lewandrowski E, et al. Myocardial injury and ventricular dysfunction related to training levels among nonelite participants in the Boston marathon. Circulation 2006;114(22):2325–33.

35. Shave R, Baggish A, George K, et al. Exercise-induced cardiac troponin elevation: evidence, mechanisms, and implications. J Am Coll Cardiol 2010;56(3):169–76.

36. 36th Bethesda Conference: eligibility recommendations for competitive athletes with cardiovascular abnormalitis. J Am Coll Cardiol 2005;45:1322–75.

37. Pelliccia A, Fagard R, Bjørnstad HH, et al. Recommendations for competitive sports participation in athletes with cardiovascular disease: a consensus document from the Study Group of Sports Cardiology of the Working Group of Cardiac Rehabilitation and Exercise Physiology and the Working Group of Myocardial and Pericardial Diseases of the European Society of Cardiology. Eur Heart J 2005;226:1422–45.

38. Elliott PM, Poloniecki J, Dickie S, et al. Sudden death in hypertrophic cardiomyopathy: identification of high risk patients. J Am Coll Cardiol 2000;36:2212–8.

39. Spirito P, Rapezzi C, Autore C, et al. Prognosis of asymptomatic patients with hypertrophic cardiomyopathy and non-sustained ventricular tachycardia. Circulation 1994;90:2743–7.

40. Monserrat L, Elliott PM, Gimeno JR, et al. Nonsustained ventricular tachycardia in hypertrophic cardiomyopathy: an independent marker of sudden death risk in young patients. J Am Coll Cardiol 2003;42:873–9.

41. Maron BJ, Savage DD, Wolfson JK, et al. Prognostic significance of 24 h ambulatory electrocardiographic monitoring in patients with hypertrophic cardiomyopathy: a prospective study. Am J Cardiol 1981;48:252–7.

42. Elliott PM, McKenna WJ. Hypertrophic cardiomyopathy. Lancet 2004;363:1881–91.

43. Adabag AS, Casey SA, Kuskowski MA, et al. Spectrum and prognostic significance of arrhythmias on ambulatory Holter electrocardiogram in hypertrophic cardiomyopathy. J Am Coll Cardiol 2005;45:697–704.

44. Bunch TJ, Chandrasekaran K, Ehrsam JE, et al. Prognostic significance of exercise induced arrhythmias and echocardiographic variables in hypertrophic cardiomyopathy. Am J Cardiol 2007;99:835–8.

45. Gimeno JR, Tomé-Esteban M, Lofiego C, et al. Exercise-induced ventricular arrhythmias and risk of sudden cardiac death in patients with hypertrophic cardiomyopathy. Eur Heart J 2009;30:2599–605.

46. Daliento L, Turrini P, Nava A, et al. Arrhythmogenic right ventricular cardiomyopathy in young versus adult patients: similarities and differences. J Am Coll Cardiol 1995;25:655–64.

47. Marcus FI, Fontaine G. Arrhythmogenic right ventricular dysplasia/cardiomyopathy: a review. Pacing Clin Electrophysiol 1995;18:1298–314.

48. Gemayel C, Pelliccia A, Thompson PD. Arrhythmogenic right ventricular cardiomyopathy. J Am Coll Cardiol 2001;38:1773–81.

49. Corrado D, Basso C, Nava A, et al. Arrhythmogenic right ventricular cardiomyopathy: current diagnostic and management strategies. Cardiol Rev 2001;9:259–65.

50. McKenna WJ, Thiene G, Nava A, et al. Task Force of the Working Group on Myocardial and Pericardial Disease of the European Society of Cardiology and of the Scientific Council on Cardiomyopathies of the International Society and Federation of Cardiology. Diagnosis of arrhythmogenic right ventricular dysplasia/cardiomyopathy. Br Heart J 1994;71:215–8.

51. Coumel P, Leenhardt A, Haddad G. Exercise ECG: prognostic implications of exercise induced arrhythmias. Pacing Clin Electrophysiol 1994;17:417–27.

52. Sequeira IB, Kirsh JA, Hamilton RM, et al. Utility of exercise testing in children and teenagers with arrhythmogenic right ventricular cardiomyopathy. Am J Cardiol 2009;104(3):411–3.

53. Bern C, Montgomery SP, Herwaldt BL, et al. Evaluation and treatment of Chagas disease in the United States. A systematic review. JAMA 2007;298:2171–81.

54. Milei J, Guerri-Guttenberg RA, Grana DR, et al. Prognostic impact of Chagas disease in the United States. Am Heart J 2009;157:22–9.

55. Dias JC, Prata A, Correia D. Problems and perspectives for Chagas disease control: in search of a realistic analysis. Rev Soc Bras Med Trop 2008;41:193–6.

56. Chiale PA, Halpern S, Nau GJ, et al. Malignant ventricular arrhythmias in chronic chagasic myocarditis. Pacing Clin Electrophysiol 1982;5:162–72.

57. Rassi A Jr, Rassi AG, Rassi SG, et al. Ventricular arrhythmias in Chagas disease. Diagnostic, prognostic and therapeutic aspects. Arq Bras Cardiol 1995;65:377–87.

58. Beckerman J, Froelicher VF. Exercise-test-induced arrhythmias: a focused review. ACC Curr J Rev 2005;12:41–4.

59. Frolkis JP, Pothier CE, Blackstone EH, et al. Frequent ventricular ectopy after exercise as a predictor of death. N Engl J Med 2003;348(9):781–90.

60. Jervell A, Lange-Nielsen F. Congenital deafmutism, functional heart disease with prolongation of the Q-T interval and sudden death. Am Heart J 1957;54(1):59–68.

61. Bianco M, Bria S, Gianfelici A, et al. Does early repolarization in the athlete have analogies with the Brugada syndrome? Eur Heart J 2001;22(6):504–10.

62. Walker J, Calkins H, Nazarian S. Evaluation of cardiac arrhythmia among athletes. Am J Med 2010;123(12):1075–81.

63. Pelliccia A, Zipes DP, Maron BJ. Bethesda Conference #36 and the European Society of Cardiology

Consensus Recommendations revisited a comparison of U.S. and European criteria for eligibility and disqualification of competitive athletes with cardiovascular abnormalities. J Am Coll Cardiol 2008; 52(24):1990–6.

64. Viskin S, Rosovski U, Sands AJ, et al. Inaccurate electrocardiographic interpretation of long QT: the majority of physicians cannot recognize a long QT when they see one. Heart Rhythm 2005;2: 569–74.

65. Kaufman ES, Priori SG, Napolitano C, et al. Electrocardiographic prediction of abnormal genotype in congenital long QT syndrome: experience in 101 related family members. J Cardiovasc Electrophysiol 2001;12:455–61.

66. Vincent GM, Timothy KW, Leppert M, et al. The spectrum of symptoms and QT intervals in carriers of the gene for the Long-QT Syndrome. N Engl J Med 1992;327:846–52.

67. Ackerman MJ, Splawski I, Makielski JC, et al. Spectrum and prevalence of cardiac sodium channel variants among black, white, Asian, and Hispanic individuals: implications for arrhythmogenic susceptibility and Brugada/long QT syndrome genetic testing. Heart Rhythm 2004;1: 600–7.

68. Wong JA, Gula LJ, Klein GJ, et al. Utility of treadmill testing in identification and genotype prediction in long-QT syndrome. Circ Arrhythm Electrophysiol 2010;3(2):120–5.

69. Takenaka K, Ai T, Shimizu W, et al. Exercise stress test amplifies genotype-phenotype correlation in the LQT1 and LQT2 forms of the Long-QT syndrome. Circulation 2003;107:838–44.

70. Pappone C, Manguso F, Santinelli R, et al. Radiofrequency ablation in children with asymptomatic Wolff–Parkinson–White syndrome. N Engl J Med 2004;351:1197–205.

71. Pappone C, Santinelli V, Rosanio S, et al. Usefulness of invasive electrophysiologic testing to stratify the risk of arrhythmic events in asymptomatic patients with Wolff–Parkinson–White pattern: results from a large prospective long-term follow-up study. J Am Coll Cardiol 2003;41:239–44.

72. Sharma AD, Yee R, Guiraudon G, et al. Sensitivity and specificity of invasive and noninvasive testing for risk of sudden death in Wolff–Parkinson–White syndrome. J Am Coll Cardiol 1987;10:373–81.

73. Wann LS, Curtis AB, January CT, et al. 2011 ACCF/AHA/HRS focused update on the management of patients with atrial fibrillation (Updating the 2006 Guideline): a report of the American College of Cardiology Foundation/American Heart Association Task Force on Practice Guidelines. J Am Coll Cardiol 2011;57(2):223.

74. Fuchs T, Torjman A, Galitzkaya L, et al. The clinical significance of ventricular arrhythmias during an exercise test in non-competitive and competitive athletes. Isr Med Assoc J 2011;13:735–9.

75. Morshedi-Meibodi A, Evans JC, Levy D, et al. Clinical correlates and prognostic significance of exercise-induced ventricular premature beats in the community: the Framingham Heart Study. Circulation 2004;109:2417–22.

76. Kennedy HL, Whitlock JA, Sprague MK, et al. Long-term follow-up of asymptomatic healthy subjects with frequent and complex ventricular ectopy. N Engl J Med 1985;312:193.

77. Elkon KB, Swerdlow TA, Myburgh DP. Persistent ventricular ectopic beats. A long-term study. S Afr Med J 1977;52:564.

78. Rodstein M, Wolloch L, Gubner RS. Mortality study of the significance of extrasystoles in an insured population. Circulation 1971;44:617.

79. Zehender M, Meinertz T, Keul J, et al. ECG variants 1. and cardiac arrhythmias in athletes: clinical relevance and rognostic importance. Am Heart J 1990; 119:1379–91.

80. Huston P, Puffer JC, MacMillan RW. The athletic heart syndrome. N Engl J Med 1985;315:24–32.

81. Viitasalo MT, Kala R, Eisalo A. Ambulatory electrocardiographic recording in endurance athletes. Br Heart J 1982;47:213–20.

82. Bjornstad H, Smith G, Storstein L, et al. Electrocardiographic and echocardiographic findings in top athletes, athletic students and sedentary controls. Cardiology 1993;82:66–74.

83. Moss AJ. Clinical significance of ventricular arrhythmias in patients with and without coronary artery disease. Prog Cardiovasc Dis 1980;23:33.

84. Bikkina M, Larson MG, Levy D. Prognostic implications of asymptomatic ventricular arrhythmias: the Framingham heart study. Ann Intern Med 1992;117:990.

85. Biffi A, Pelliccia A, Verdile L, et al. Long-term clinical significance of frequent ventricular tachyarrhythmias in trained athletes. J Am Coll Cardiol 2002;40:446–52.

86. Biffi A, Maron BJ, DiGiacinto B, et al. Relation between training-induced left ventricular hypertrophy and risk of ventricular tachyarrhythmias in elite athletes. Am J Cardiol 2008;101:1792–5.

87. McHenry PL, Fisch C, Jordan JW, et al. Cardiac arrhythmias observed during maximal treadmill exercise testing in clinically normal men. Am J Cardiol 1972;29:331–6.

88. Marieb MA, Beller GA, Gibson RS, et al. Clinical relevance of exercise-induced ventricular arrhythmias in suspected coronary artery disease. Am J Cardiol 1990;66:172–8.

89. Schweikert RA, Pashkow FJ, Snader CE, et al. Association of exercise-induced ventricular ectopic activity with thallium myocardial perfusion and angiographic coronary artery disease in stable, low-risk populations. Am J Cardiol 1999;83:530–4.

90. Faris JV, McHenry PL, Jordan JW, et al. Prevalence and reproducibility of exercise-induced ventricular arrhythmias during maximal exercise testing in normal men. Am J Cardiol 1976;37:617–22.

91. Beckerman J, Mathur A, Stahr S, et al. Exercise-induced ventricular arrhythmias and cardiovascular death. Ann Noninvasive Electrocardiol 2005; 10(1):47–52.

92. Weiner DA, Levine SR, Klein MD, et al. Ventricular arrhythmias during exercise testing: mechanism, response to coronary bypass surgery, and prognostic significance. Am J Cardiol 1984;53:1553–7.

93. McHenry PL, Morris SN, Kavalier M, et al. Comparative study of exercise-induced ventricular arrhythmias in normal subjects and patients with documented coronary artery disease. Am J Cardiol 1976;37:609–16.

94. Partington S, Myers J, Cho S, et al. Prevalence and prognostic value of exercise-induced ventricular arrhythmias. Am Heart J 2003;145:139–46.

95. Sami M, Chaitman B, Fisher L, et al. Significance of exercise-induced ventricular arrhythmia in stable coronary artery disease: a Coronary Artery Surgery Study project. Am J Cardiol 1984;54:1182–8.

96. Casella G, Pavesi PC, Sangiorgio P, et al. Exercise-induced ventricular arrhythmias in patients with healed myocardial infarction. Int J Cardiol 1993; 40:229–35.

97. Udall JA, Ellestad MH. Predictive implications of ventricular premature contractions associated with treadmill stress testing. Circulation 1977;56:985–9.

98. Jouven X, Zureik M, Desnos M, et al. Long-term outcome in asymptomatic men with exercise-induced premature ventricular depolarizations. N Engl J Med 2000;343:826–33.

99. Coumel P, Fidelle J, Lucet V, et al. Catecholamine-induced severe ventricular arrhythmias with Adam-Stokes in children: report of four cases. Br Heart J 1978;40:28–37.

100. Leenhardt A, Lucet V, Denjoy I, et al. Catecholaminergic polymorphic ventricular tachycardia in children: a 7-year follow-up of 21 patients. Circulation 1995;91:1512–9.

101. Priori SG, Napolitano C, Tiso N, et al. Mutations in the cardiac ryanodine receptor gene (hRyR2) underlie catecholaminergic polymorphic ventricular tachycardia. Circulation 2001;103:196–200.

102. Lahat H, Pras E, Olender T, et al. A missense mutation in a highly conserved region of CASQ2 is associated with autosomal recessive catecholamine-induced polymorphic ventricular tachycardia in Bedouin families from Israel. Am J Hum Genet 2001;69:1378–84.

103. Priori SG, Napolitano C, Memmi M, et al. Clinical and molecular characterization of patients with catecholaminergic polymorphic ventricular tachycardia. Circulation 2002;106:69–74.

104. Watanabe H, Chopra N, Laver D, et al. Flecainide prevents catecholaminergic polymorphic ventricular tachycardia in mice and humans. Nat Med 2009;15:380–3.

105. Hayashi M, Denjoy I, Extramiana F, et al. Incidence and risk factors of arrhythmic events in catecholaminergic polymorphic ventricular tachycardia. Circulation 2009;119:2426–34.

106. Sofi F, Capalbo A, Pucci N, et al. Cardiovascular evaluation, including resting and exercise electrocardiography, before participation in competitive sports: cross sectional study. BMJ 2008;337(7661):88–92.

107. Gibbons RJ, Balady GJ, Bricker JT, et al. ACC/AHA 2002 guideline update for exercise testing: summary article: a report of the American College of Cardiology/American Heart Association Task Force on Practice Guidelines (Committee to Update the 1997 Exercise Testing Guidelines) ACC/AHA 2002 guideline update for exercise testing: summary article. Circulation 2002;106:1883–92.

108. Myers J, Froelicher VF. Optimizing the exercise test for pharmacological investigations. Circulation 1990;82(5):1839–46.

109. Furtado EC, Araujp CG. Cardiac arrhythmias triggered by sudden and dynamic efforts. Ann Noninvasive Electrocardiol 2010;15(2):151–6.

110. Young DZ, Lampert S, Graboys TB, et al. Safety of maximal exercise testing in patients at high risk for ventricular arrhythmia. Circulation 1984; 70(2):184–91.

Leisure-time Physical Activity and Sport Participation in Patients with Cardiomyopathies

Antonio Pelliccia, MD*, Filippo M. Quattrini, MD, PhD

KEYWORDS

• Cardiomyopathies • Sudden cardiac arrest • Exercise training • Sport activity

KEY POINTS

- Scientific evidence suggests that subjects affected by cardiomyopathies are at increased risk of sudden cardiac arrest usually in association with exercise training and competitive sport activity.
- Physicians are faced with the task to advise patients with cardiomyopathies how to combine the benefits of an active lifestyle without incurring the risk for adverse cardiac events.
- Physicians have an ethical, medical, and legal obligation to exhaustively inform the patient with cardiomyopathy of the risks inherent to exercise training and athletic lifestyle and, when the risk for cardiac deterioration or cardiac arrest seems to be likely, to advise withdrawing from sport.
- It seems reasonable that the potential risk of exercise training should not deny to the large proportion of patients affected by cardiomyopathies the many cardiovascular benefits offered by regular exercise.
- The current recommendations provide the basis for risk stratification and management of patients with cardiomyopathies who want to practice physical activity and offer to physicians updated knowledge for appropriate exercise prescription.

INTRODUCTION

Regular physical activity is advised as therapeutic procedure for several cardiovascular (CV) and metabolic diseases and represents a major determinant for reducing the burden of CV risk.[1,2] Indeed, exercise programs and participation in sport events have become hallmarks of lifestyle in Western populations, including an increasing proportion of individuals with inherited or acquired pathologic cardiac conditions.

Increasing scientific evidence[3–6] suggests, however, that individuals with underlying (even clinically silent) CV disease have an increased risk for clinical deterioration and sudden cardiac death (SCD) in relation to their participation in exercise programs and sport competitions. Therefore, the demand for an active lifestyle by individuals with CV diseases represents a challenging decision for the physician, who faces the dilemma of how to promote the benefits of an active lifestyle without incurring the risk for adverse cardiac events. The physician is thus required to have adequate knowledge regarding prescription of the type, intensity, and frequency of exercise programs that expose the patient with cardiac disease to the lowest risk of clinical deterioration or cardiac arrest.

Disclosures: No conflict of interest to declare.
Institute of Sports Medicine and Science, Rome, Italy
* Corresponding author. Institute of Sports Medicine and Science, Largo Piero Gabrielli 1, Rome 00197, Italy.
E-mail address: ant.pelliccia@libero.it

Card Electrophysiol Clin 5 (2013) 65–71
http://dx.doi.org/10.1016/j.ccep.2012.11.005
1877-9182/13/$ – see front matter © 2013 Elsevier Inc. All rights reserved.

THE RISK OF EXERCISE AND SPORT IN PATIENTS WITH CARDIOMYOPATHIES

The major risk for young individuals with arrhythmogenic cardiomyopathies (CMPs) (eg, hypertrophic CMP [HCM]) is related to occurrence of ventricular fibrillation, ultimately leading to cardiac arrest. This event is unpredictable, and commonly happens in the absence of prior symptoms.[5–11] However, several reports suggest that cardiac arrest in young patients with CMPs more commonly occurs on the athletic field and in relation to physical activity.[7–11] Although no conclusive evidence demonstrates the independent role of exercise and sport, several observations support the concept that intense exercise training may be primarily responsible for triggering ventricular arrhythmias leading to SCD.[7–13] Indeed, in adolescents and young adults participating in vigorous physical exertion and competitive sport, Corrado and colleagues[13] demonstrated a 2.8 increase in relative risk for sudden death compared with nonathletic control subjects.

The mechanisms explaining the increased susceptibility to ventricular arrhythmias in patients with CMPs are related to the combined action of neurohormonal changes induced by the exercise (eg, increased adrenergic output to heart, associated with increased myocardial oxygen consumption, and fluid and electrolyte imbalance) in the presence of structural cardiac abnormalities (including patched intramyocardial fibrosis and myocardial disarray, and small coronary artery media thickening) (**Fig. 1**). Therefore, exercise acts as a trigger for ventricular arrhythmias in susceptible individuals with underlying (even unrecognized) structural cardiac abnormalities.[8,13]

Indirect evidence for the proarrhythmic role of intensive exercise training is offered by the observation that young athletes with frequent and sustained ventricular arrhythmias show a substantial reduction in frequency and complexity (or even disappearance) of the arrhythmias after a short (average, 3 months) period of complete detraining.[14] Subsequent resumption of physical activity and sport participation is, indeed, associated with recurrence of the arrhythmias, although less clinically relevant.[15] These observations support the decision by a medical practice to withdraw susceptible individuals with HCM (and other CMPs) from intense exercise and sport participation to reduce the actual risk for cardiac arrest.[16–18] Indeed, patients with HCM disqualified from competitive sport incurred no death or clinical deterioration over a long-term follow-up.[19]

RECOMMENDATIONS FOR LEISURE-TIME PHYSICAL ACTIVITY AND SPORT PARTICIPATION

To help physicians address the difficult problem of prescribing physical activity and sport participation in young and adult individuals with CMPs, specific recommendations have been released.[16–18,20]

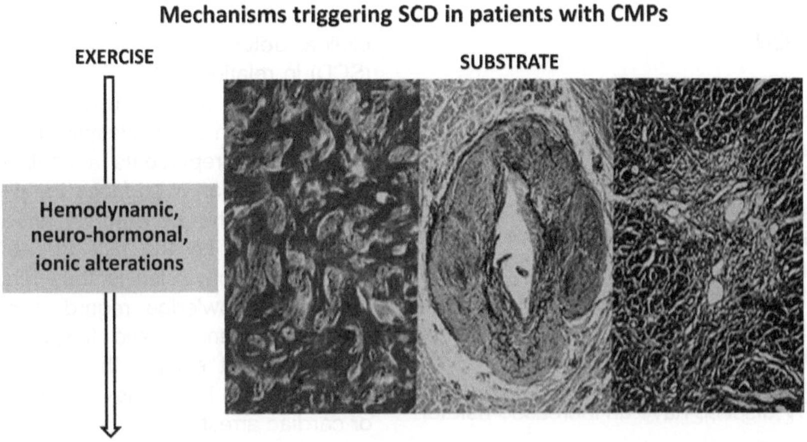

Mechanisms triggering SCD in patients with CMPs

Fig. 1. Schematic representation of the mechanisms leading to sudden death in patients with cardiomyopathies in association with exercise training. Exercise acts as a trigger for arrhythmias through increased hemodynamic load, associated with increased adrenergic output to the heart and possibly ion imbalance, in the presence of underlying structural abnormalities including myocardial disarray, extensive interstitial fibrosis, and small vessel disease (causing ischemia). These alterations represent the background for electrical instability and fragmentation of the electrical wave-front, triggering ventricular arrhythmias potentially degenerating into VF and cardiac arrest. VF, Ventricular Fibrillation.

These recommendations assume that diagnosis of CMP has already been made, so that the issues directly related to screening are not discussed in this article.

The current recommendations represent the consensus document of an international panel of experts and are based on scientific evidence, when available, and on personal experience and consensus of experts in most instances. However, in consideration of the scarcity of scientific investigations concerning the effect of regular exercise training and sport activities on the clinical course of most CMPs, caution in applying these recommendations is needed and efforts should be made to tailor precise advice to each patient.

ROLE OF THE EXAMINING PHYSICIAN

The role of the examining physician is to provide careful assessment and offer appropriate advice regarding the exercise program and sport activity and, when the case, appropriate treatment of the candidate with CMPs. The physician should have in mind that, although vigorous exercise and competitive sport may increase the risk for an adverse event, the benefits of regular physical activity by far outweigh the dangers.

At first, the physician should carefully research subtle symptoms in physically active individuals. Several subjects dying suddenly during exercise had reported previous symptoms, often misinterpreted, that had not raised medical attention. The patient should also be informed that vigorous exercise per se does not exclude the presence of a serious CV condition and high levels of performance do not guarantee against incidence of cardiac events.

The physician has the ethical, medical, and legal obligation to exhaustively inform the candidate of the risks inherent to exercise training and athletic lifestyle, based on scientific evidence and prudent recommendations.[16–18,20] When the risk for cardiac deterioration or cardiac arrest seems to be very possible, the physician should suggest the patient with CMP withdraw from exercise training and sport. This recommendation is particularly true in case of competitive sport activities. Because of the unique structure and pressures of competitive sports, individuals with CMPs (and other CV diseases) may not always retain an unbiased, objective approach in assessing the overall risk associated with an athletic lifestyle. The recommendations are intended, therefore, to support the physician's decision in such difficult scenarios and offer protection to patients with CMP from the unsustainable hazard of competitive sports.

PRESCRIPTION OF LEISURE-TIME PHYSICAL ACTIVITY IN PATIENTS WITH CMPS

For the purpose of this article, recreational sports activities are defined in juxtaposition to competitive sports and refer to a wide range of physical activities, from modest to vigorous in intensity, performed either in a regular or inconsistent basis not requiring systematic training or pursuit of excellence, nor involving the same psychological pressure to surpass other participants, which is characteristic of competitive sports.

The clinician is frequently confronted with the request of designing leisure-time exercise programs for young individuals with HCM or other CMPs who do not aspire to organized sports participation (or have been withdrawn or disqualified from competitive sports), but aspire to maintain a physically active lifestyle.

At present, the risk of habitual noncompetitive physical activities in young and adult patients with genetically transmitted cardiac diseases is undefined. Despite the paucity of scientific evidence in this area, it is likely that a certain degree of risk will remain associated with participation even in amateur and leisure-time physical activities. However, it seems reasonable that the potential risk of exercise should not deprive a large proportion of patients with HCM and other genetic cardiac diseases of the many CV benefits afforded by regular exercise.[20]

It is necessary for the clinician to individualize exercise prescription, balancing the clinical status of the patient with the physical activity under consideration. To the scope, the physician should be aware of the peculiarities of the HCM (or other CMP) in the candidate and assess the overall risk profile. Criteria for risk assessment in the different CMPs are beyond the scope of this article; however, for the purpose of exercise prescription the physician should consider the following criteria, which reasonably indicate a "low risk":

- Lack of sudden death among first-degree relatives
- Relatively "mild" structural abnormalities. For example, in HCM the left ventricular wall thickness ≤18 mm; transverse left atrium diameter <45 mm; no evidence of gadolinium late-enhancement on cardiac magnetic resonance (CMR).
- Mild left ventricular dysfunction. For example, in HCM absence of left ventricular outflow tract obstruction, and normal or only mildly impaired left ventricular diastolic function. In dilated CMP (DCM), mild systolic dysfunction (ejection fraction $\geq45\%$)

- Normal or near-normal hemodynamic behavior during exercise testing (ie, normal increase in blood pressure)
- Lack of significant supraventricular arrhythmias (supraventricular tachycardia or atrial fibrillation) and ventricular arrhythmias (non-sustained ventricular tachycardia) documented at the exercise testing or 24-hour electrocardiogram monitoring

When all these conditions are satisfied, implying a "low risk" CMP, the physician can reassure the patient with respect to the capability to sustain a regular exercise program without major limitations. The indication for the type of exercise may ultimately be liberal, and can address more closely the patient's aspirations, even including those characterized by moderate- to high-intensity exercise programs. However, when one or more of the previously mentioned criteria of risk are present, the physician more cautiously should prescribe physical activities selected among those with moderate and low intensity, and less likely to induce arrhythmias.

Types of physical activity that may be advised to patients with CMPs after assessment of the risk profile are here schematically identified as high-intensity, moderate-intensity, and low-intensity and reported in **Table 1**. In all cases, a periodic control should be advised, usually on an annual basis, to evaluate the progression of the disease and any change in the clinical picture requiring adjustment to the individual exercise profile.

MODALITY OF LEISURE-TIME PHYSICAL ACTIVITY

In addition, it is important to express specific recommendations about modality of exercise programs that may reduce the arrhythmic risk in patients with CMPs. First, patients should start an exercise session with a warm-up period and specifically avoid explosive exertion, characterized by short time, high-intensity exercise. At the end of the session, an appropriate cool-down period is also recommended.

Second, exercise programs (even if recreational in nature) that imply progressive levels of intensity and lead to higher levels of conditioning should be closely monitored by the physician, in contact with the coach. Third, the patient should avoid exercise in extremely adverse environmental conditions, including very hot, humid, or very cold weather. In these circumstances exercise sessions should be performed in indoor facilities where appropriate temperature is maintained.

Fourth, patients who suffered impaired consciousness (eg, syncope and near-syncope) are subject to considerably higher risk for traumatic injury while engaged in sports, and such activities as diving, rock climbing, motorcycling, and bench-pressing maneuvers should be prudently

Table 1 Classification of physical activities in relation to the estimated intensity of exercise[a]		
High-Intensity	**Moderate-Intensity**	**Low-Intensity**
Basketball	Cross-country skiing (flat course)	Archery
Baseball	Horseback riding[b]	Bowling
Boxing[b]	Jogging	Brisk walking
Circuit weight-training	Moderate-intensity weights	Cricket
Cross-country skiing	Sailing[d]	Gymnastics
Ice hockey[b,c]	Stationary rowing	Golfing
Road cycling[b,c]	Swimming[d]	Moderate hiking
Rowing/canoeing[c]	Tennis (doubles)	Skating[c]
Running[c]	Volleyball	Shooting
Soccer		Stationary bicycle
Tennis (singles)		Treadmill
Track events		Low-intensity weights
Wrestling[b]		
Windsurfing[d]		

[a] Activities to be prudentially avoided in patients with cardiomyopathies are those performed in dangerous environments (eg, rock climbing, scuba diving) or associated with increased life-threatening risk if syncope occurs (eg, motorcycling, auto racing).
[b] These sports involve the potential for traumatic injury, which should be taken into consideration for individuals at risk of impaired consciousness or with an implanted cardioverter-defibrillator.
[c] Is intended as individual sporting activity and not as member of a team.
[d] The possibility of impaired consciousness occurring during water-related activities should be taken into account with respect to the clinical profile of the individual patient.

avoided. Finally, individuals with an implanted cardioverter-defibrillator (ICD) should avoid contact sports because of risk of body collision with traumatic injury or inappropriate discharge. However, presence of an implanted ICD does not represent, per se, restriction from amateur, leisure-time physical activity after individual assessment.[20]

EDUCATION OF THE PATIENT

The final organization of the exercise program ultimately depends on the interaction between physician and patient. Patient education is, therefore, important. The patient should be fully informed of the clinical peculiarities and the risk profile of the disease, and warned about the symptoms and signs that may potentially occur in association with exercise.

The clinician should teach a patient participating in individual sport activities (eg, jogging, running, canoeing, or skiing) to take control over the level of exertion by assessing heart rate (devices assessing heart rate are commercially available and efficient in monitoring heart rate) and to be aware of any change in the clinical status.

Patients participating in a recreational team sport (eg, soccer, volleyball, or basketball) should be informed to take a voluntary a break, or to ask the coach for a turnover, in case the intensity or duration of exercise may become disproportionate to the recommendations stated by the physician.

Finally, it is wise for patients with arrhythmogenic CMPs to be aware of and ask about the presence of an automatic defibrillator in the gym or sport facility where they are going to exercise. Availability of such a device may represent a criterion for the choice of the most convenient facility in which to perform exercise.

Occasionally, the decision regarding the structure of exercise programs may be influenced by legal responsibility of the physician, or the possibility that recommendations may be (deliberately) ignored by the patient, or the perception that the cardiac risk will be considered unsustainable by the family. In these cases, particular caution is requested and the physician's recommendations should be structured on an individual basis.

PHYSICAL EDUCATION CLASS IN YOUNG PATIENTS WITH CMPS

Questions related to participation in recreational exercise often arise with regard to compulsory physical education classes in elementary or junior high school. Many components of such classes may be truly recreational and clearly cannot be regarded as competitive in nature. It is suggested that parents in concert with school officials and their physician undertake a review of physical education class requirements (type, duration, and frequency of exercise programs) and a decision relative to participation in physical education class should be individualized as much as possible. However, in consideration of the relevance of social and educational aspects of physical exercise in school for children and young individuals, it is highly recommended to avoid unnecessary medical prohibition for participation in physical education class.[20]

COMPETITIVE SPORT PARTICIPATION IN PATIENTS WITH CMPS

For the purpose of this article, competitive and professional sports activities are defined in juxtaposition to leisure-time activities and indicate a wide range of sport disciplines, from modest to vigorous in intensity, performed on a regular basis and requiring systematic training, with the aim to pursue excellence in competition, usually involving psychological pressure to surpass other participants.

Competitive and professional athletes participate in official competitions (either local, regional, national, or international), such as team or individual sports events that, placing a high premium on excellence and achievement, are organized and scheduled in the agenda of recognized athletic associations. Characteristic of competitive sports is the strong proclivity for participants to exert themselves physically until their limits and enhance performance. In this context, competitive athletes (in particular, the elite and professional) represent a special subset of active population, not only for their superior performances, but also for the large visibility and substantial economic interests they gather and the intense pressure to which they are exposed by sponsors, media, and athletic associations. In several countries the participation in competitive and professional sport is regulated by rules, including also the need for medical clearance (with certification of eligibility), to the individual willing to enter the competitive athletic career.

These considerations have prompted scientific associations (American Heart Association, American College of Cardiology, and European Society of Cardiology [ESC]) to provide recommendations for competitive sport participation by individuals with cardiac disease including CMPs.[16–18] The rationale for offering an expert consensus document concerning participation in competitive sports in individuals with CMPs is based on the widely accepted clinical perception, substantiated by scientific evidence, that athletes with underlying (even clinically silent) CMPs have an increased risk for SCD or clinical deterioration.[21]

The existing recommendations (either Bethesda Conference [BC] #36 or the ESC) agree that patients with arrhythmogenic CMPs should be restricted from participation in competitive sport. This advice is based on the awareness that the arrhythmic risk of individuals with CMPs is not completely quantifiable and occurrence of fatal arrhythmias may be the first sign of disease. Therefore, in view of the unpredictable arrhythmic risk, the American Heart Association and ESC recommendations suggest a high degree of prudence, and specifically state that "Individuals with a definite diagnosis of HCM, DCM and ARVC should not participate in any competitive sports activities."[16]

One possible exception is represented, after careful evaluation, by subjects with HCM or DCM considered at "low risk," according to the previously mentioned criteria. For these subjects eligibility for competitions can be granted on an individual basis for low-intensity sports (see **Table 1**) (eg, archery, golf, shooting) based on the assumption that participation in these activities has no, or only unremarkable, impact on the clinical outcome of the disease. Major caution is needed for patients with definite diagnosis of arrhythmogenic right ventricular cardiomyopathy (ARVC), in which the arrhythmic risk inherent to the disease is unpredictable.[16,17]

SPECIAL CONSIDERATIONS

The placement of an ICD does not change the recommendations; restriction from participation in competitive sports is advisable, because engagement in regular training and competition might impact adversely the natural history of the disease. The presence of a free-standing automated external defibrillator at sporting events should not be considered either absolute protection against sudden death or treatment strategy for known CMPs, or a justification for participation in competitive sports in patients with previously diagnosed diseases.[16–18]

REFERENCES

1. Fletcher GF, Balady G, Blair SN, et al. Statement on exercise: benefits and recommendations for physical activity programs for all Americans. A statement for health professionals by the Committee on Exercise and Cardiac Rehabilitation of the Council on Clinical Cardiology, American Heart Association. Circulation 1996;94:857–62.

2. Thompson PD, Buchner D, Pina IL, et al. Exercise and physical activity in the prevention and treatment of atherosclerotic cardiovascular disease: a statement from the Council on Clinical Cardiology (Subcommittee on Exercise, Rehabilitation, and Prevention) and the Council on Nutrition, Physical Activity, and Metabolism (Subcommittee on Physical Activity). Circulation 2003;107:3109–16.

3. Siscovick DS, Weiss NS, Fletcher RH, et al. The incidence of primary cardiac arrest during vigorous exercise. N Engl J Med 1984;311:874–7.

4. Mittleman MA, Maclure M, Tofler GH, et al. Triggering of acute myocardial infarction by heavy physical exertion. Protection against triggering by regular exertion. Determinants of Myocardial Infarction Onset Study Investigators. N Engl J Med 1993; 329:1677–83.

5. Van Camp SP, Bloor CM, Mueller FO, et al. Nontraumatic sports death in high school and college athletes. Med Sci Sports Exerc 1995;27:641–7.

6. Burke AP, Farb V, Virmani R, et al. Sports-related and non-sports-related sudden cardiac death in young adults. Am Heart J 1991;121:568–75.

7. Maron BJ. Sudden death in young athletes: lessons from the Hank Gathers affair. N Engl J Med 1993; 329:55–7.

8. Maron BJ, Shirani J, Poliac LC, et al. Sudden death in young competitive athletes. Clinical, demographic, and pathological profiles. JAMA 1996; 276:199–204.

9. Maron BJ. Cardiovascular risks to young persons on the athletic field. Ann Intern Med 1998;129:379–86.

10. Maron BJ, Mitten MJ, Quandt EF, et al. Competitive athletes with cardiovascular disease—the case of Nicholas Knapp. N Engl J Med 1998;339:1632–5.

11. Maron BJ, Gohman TE, Aeppli D. Prevalence of sudden cardiac death during competitive sports activities in Minnesota high school athletes. J Am Coll Cardiol 1998;32:1881–4.

12. Thompson PD, Franklin BA, Balady GJ, et al. Exercise and acute cardiovascular events, placing the risks into perspective: a scientific statement from the American Heart Association Council on Nutrition, Physical Activity, and Metabolism and the Council on Clinical Cardiology. Circulation 2007; 115:2358–68.

13. Corrado D, Basso C, Rizzoli G, et al. Does sport activity enhance the risk of sudden death in adolescents and young adults? J Am Coll Cardiol 2003;42: 1959–63.

14. Biffi A, Maron BJ, Verdile L, et al. Impact of physical deconditioning on ventricular tachyarrhythmias in trained athletes. J Am Coll Cardiol 2004;44: 1053–8.

15. Biffi A, Maron BJ, Culasso F, et al. Patterns of ventricular tachyarrhythmias associated with training, deconditioning and retraining in elite

athletes without cardiovascular abnormalities. Am J Cardiol 2011;107:697–703.

16. Maron BJ, Zipes DP. 36th Bethesda Conference. Eligibility recommendations for competitive athletes with cardiovascular abnormalities. J Am Coll Cardiol 2005;45:1312–75.

17. Pelliccia A, Fagard R, Bjørnstad HH, et al. Recommendations for competitive sports participation in athletes with cardiovascular disease. Eur Heart J 2005;26:1422–45.

18. Pelliccia A, Corrado D, Bjornstad HH, et al. Recommendations for participation in competitive sport and leisure-time physical activity in individuals with cardiomyopathies, myocarditis and pericarditis. Eur J Cardiovasc Prev Rehabil 2006;13: 876–85.

19. Corrado D, Basso C, Schiavon M, et al. Screening for hypertrophic cardiomyopathy in young athletes. N Engl J Med 1998;339:364–9.

20. Maron BJ, Chaitman BR, Ackerman MJ, et al. Recommendations for physical activity and recreational sports participation for young patients with genetic cardiovascular diseases. Circulation 2004; 109:2807–16.

21. Maron BJ, Maron MS. Hypertrophic cardiomyopathy. Lancet 2012. [Epub ahead of print].

ST-Segment Elevation and Sudden Death in the Athlete

Alessandro Zorzi, MD[a], Mohamed ElMaghawry, MD[a,b],
Federico Migliore, MD[a], Ilaria Rigato, MD, PhD[a],
Cristina Basso, MD, PhD[c], Gaetano Thiene, MD[c],
Domenico Corrado, MD, PhD[a,*]

KEYWORDS

- Athlete • J wave • ST segment • Brugada syndrome • Sudden death • Ventricular fibrillation

KEY POINTS

- A minority of sudden deaths in young athletes is caused by primary electrical diseases, such as the Brugada syndrome and idiopathic ventricular fibrillation.
- The early-repolarization electrocardiogram (ECG) pattern is traditionally considered benign; however, an association between some variants of early repolarization and idiopathic ventricular fibrillation has been recently reported (so-called early repolarization syndrome).
- The Brugada syndrome and the early repolarization syndrome may represent different phenotypic expressions of a common physiopathologic mechanism. The term J-wave syndromes has been coined to group together these 2 conditions, characterized by J-point elevation and ventricular arrhythmias.
- The Brugada ECG pattern is rare among athletes and is associated with an increased risk of sudden death, whereas the early-repolarization ECG pattern is very common and raises the odds of experiencing idiopathic ventricular fibrillation only minimally.

SUDDEN DEATH IN ATHLETES WITH APPARENTLY NORMAL HEARTS: ROLE OF THE J-WAVE SYNDROMES

In most cases of malignant ventricular arrhythmias or sudden death, a structural cardiac abnormality is evidenced by clinical investigations or autopsy. In senior athletes sudden deaths during physical activity usually occur as arrhythmic complications of an acute coronary syndrome, whereas other cardiovascular disorders, such as cardiomyopathies, congenital heart diseases, or myocarditis, account for the majority of fatal events among younger sportsmen.[1]

Sometimes sudden death occurs with an apparently normal heart on standard clinical evaluation or autopsy investigation. Inability to detect structural abnormalities may depend on the unknown or concealed nature of the underlying pathologic substrate, along with the low sensitivity of currently available tests. Subtle structural heart conditions at risk of arrhythmic sudden death include coronary artery spasm superimposed on a nonobstructive atherosclerotic plaque, focal myocarditis, or segmental cardiomyopathies. The ultimate diagnosis of these structural lesions may require invasive clinical investigations, such as endocardial voltage mapping and endomyocardial biopsy, or

Disclosures: No conflicts of interest to declare.
Sources of funding: This study was supported by Fondazione Cariparo, Padova and Rovigo, Italy; and Registry of Cardio-Cerebro-Vascular Pathology, Veneto Region, Venice, Italy.
[a] Division of Cardiology, Department of Cardiac, Thoracic and Vascular Sciences, University of Padova, Via Giustiniani 2, 35120, Padova, Italy; [b] Department of Cardiology, Aswan Heart Centre, Kasr El Hajjar Street, PO Box 81512, Aswan, Egypt; [c] Cardiovascular Pathology, Department of Cardiac, Thoracic and Vascular Sciences, University of Padova, Via A. Gabelli 61, 35121, Padova, Italy
* Corresponding author. Division of Cardiology, Department of Cardiac, Thoracic and Vascular Sciences, University of Padova, Via Giustiniani 2, 35120, Padova, Italy.
E-mail address: domenico.corrado@unipd.it

cardiacEP.theclinics.com

postmortem histologic analysis. In fact, large autopsy series indicate that macroscopic heart features are normal in nearly one-third of sudden deaths in young people and athletes, but in the majority histologic study unmasks the pathologic substrate. However, a minority of sudden death victims have neither macroscopic nor microscopic evidence of structural heart disease: the cause of these fatalities is probably a primary electrical disease (ion-channel diseases or channelopathies), including long-QT and short-QT syndrome, catecholaminergic polymorphic ventricular tachycardia, Brugada syndrome, or idiopathic ventricular fibrillation.[2–6]

Brugada syndrome is characterized by the association of ST-segment elevation at the J point in the right precordial leads V1 to V3 and ventricular arrhythmias.[7,8] Recently it has been reported that J-point elevation in the inferolateral leads is also associated with an increased risk of idiopathic ventricular fibrillation and cardiovascular death (so-called early repolarization syndrome).[9–22] Because of their common electrophysiologic bases and clinical features, the Brugada syndrome and the early repolarization syndrome may represent a continuous spectrum of phenotypic expression, termed J-wave syndromes, although they differ with respect to the magnitude and location of leads in abnormal J-point elevation.[23,24]

In the setting of preparticipation screening, appropriate differential diagnosis between physiologic and pathologic ST-segment elevation is of utmost importance not only to prevent sport-related sudden deaths but also to avoid unnecessary disqualification from competition for changes that fall within the normal range for athletes.[25] This article addresses the potential relationship between ST-segment elevation and the risk of sudden death during sports. In addition, the differential diagnosis between malignant ST-segment elevation and benign early repolarization associated with "athlete's heart" is discussed.

MECHANISMS UNDERLYING ST-SEGMENT ELEVATION AND ARRHYTHMOGENESIS

The action potential of the epicardium physiologically shows a more prominent transient outward current (I_{to})-mediated phase-1 notch than that of the endocardium. Experimental studies demonstrated that this transmural difference in the early phases of the action potential gives rise to the electrocardiographic pattern of early repolarization: that is, QRS slurring or ST-segment elevation at the J point (Fig. 1).[26] An increase in net repolarizing currents, caused either by a decrease of inward currents (such as the Na^+ sodium current or the L-type calcium currents) or enhancement of outward currents (such as the I_{to} or adenosine triphosphate–sensitive potassium currents), leads to augmentation of the dispersion of repolarization and accentuation of ST-segment elevation.[27–29] In canine right ventricular wedge preparations, acetylcholine depresses the epicardial but not the endocardial action-potential plateau, by suppressing the calcium current and/or augmenting the potassium current, and leads to an upsloping and concave ST-segment elevation, which is readily reversed with atropine (Fig. 2).[26,30] This process explains the prominent early-repolarization pattern observed at rest in highly trained athletes with marked vagotonia adaptation. Although acetylcholine alone is capable of causing loss of the action-potential dome in isolated right ventricular epicardial tissues, these changes are unlikely to provoke phase-2 reentry and ventricular arrhythmias in healthy individuals unless external factors, such as hypothermia or myocardial ischemia, accentuate the dispersion of repolarization.[30,31]

Genetically determined ion-channel defects that accentuate the phase-1 notch in the epicardial action potential represent the physiopathologic basis of Brugada syndrome (see Fig. 1). In fact, if the outward shift of currents is pathologically increased to a more negative potential, the action-potential dome is lost, giving rise to an electrocardiogram (ECG) pattern consisting of marked J-point elevation with downsloping and coved-type ST-segment elevation (type-1 Brugada ECG pattern). Loss of function in the SCN5A gene encoding for the cardiac sodium channel has been discovered in up to 25% of patients with Brugada syndrome.[32,33] The genetic defect causes a net augmentation of the repolarizing current and appearance of a markedly elevated J point. Because of the intrinsic differences of I_{to} density in different myocardial regions, such loss of the action-potential dome is usually heterogeneous, resulting in marked abbreviation of action potential at some sites but not others. The most prominent changes are observed in the right ventricular outflow tract, explored by the ECG leads V1 to V2, which usually disclose the Brugada ECG pattern in affected individuals. Propagation of the action-potential dome from sites at which it is still maintained to sites at which it is abolished may lead to local reexcitation (so-called phase-2 reentry) and development of closely coupled extrasystoles (R-on-T phenomenon) triggering ventricular fibrillation. External factors that worsen the epicardial-endocardial heterogeneity of repolarization, such as hypokalemia, hypothermia, and administration of class-I antiarrhythmic drugs

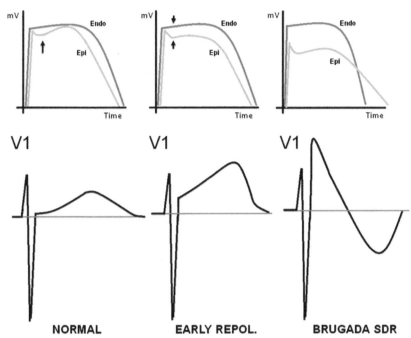

Fig. 1. Simultaneous records of the epicardial and endocardial myocyte action potentials (*top*) and electrocardiographic pattern in lead V1 (*bottom*). The effect of acetylcholine accentuates the physiologic notch at the beginning of the plateau (phase 1) on the epicardial but not endocardial action potential, giving rise to a transmural voltage gradient that manifests as J point and ST-segment elevation (so-called early repolarization). A genetic defect in the sodium channel increases the outward shift of currents to a more negative potential so that the epicardial action potential dome is lost. This mechanism gives rise to a coved-type ST-segment elevation followed by a negative T wave in the surface electrocardiogram (type 1 Brugada electrocardiogram pattern). SDR, syndrome.

and acetylcholine, may facilitate the occurrence of ventricular arrhythmias.[23,26,27]

A lesser accentuation of the epicardial action-potential notch, with preservation of the dome, is associated with a smaller prolongation of the right ventricular epicardial action potential; this represents the electrophysiologic basis of the saddleback (types 2 and 3) Brugada ECG patterns (**Fig. 3**). In Brugada patients, transition from saddleback to coved ST-segment elevation may occur either spontaneously, as a consequence of autonomic changes (**Fig. 4**), or after administration of sodium-channel blockers such as procainamide, pilsicainide, propafenone, flecainide, and disopyramide. By contrast, quinidine, which inhibits the I_{to}, reduces the magnitude of the J wave and normalizes ST-segment elevation.[34–36]

RIGHT PRECORDIAL ST-SEGMENT ELEVATION AND THE BRUGADA SYNDROME

First described in 1992, Brugada syndrome is a genetically determined disease, characterized by typical electrocardiographic signs and propensity to sudden death secondary to polymorphic ventricular tachycardia or ventricular fibrillation in the absence of structural heart disease.[8] Its estimated prevalence ranges from 1 to 5 per 10,000 individuals in Europe to 12 per 10,000 inhabitants in Southeast Asia.[37–39] It is characterized by a higher prevalence among males (approximately 80% of patients) and variable penetrance, resulting in a high number of genetically affected family members presenting with a concealed form of disease. The mean age at diagnosis is 40 to 45 years and most of the arrhythmic events also take place at that age, mainly during sleep or rest, or after large meals. The syndrome is responsible for 4% of all sudden deaths and for up to 20% of sudden deaths in patients without structural heart disease. It is also known as Lai Tai (Thailand), Bangungot (Philippines), and Pokkuri (Japan), and there is evidence linking Brugada syndrome to sudden infant death syndrome.[40]

Clinically, syncope and cardiac arrest are the most common manifestations of Brugada syndrome. These events usually occur during sleep or at rest, and rarely during sports activity. Fever and the use of certain medications may exacerbate the manifestations of Brugada syndrome.[41,42] However, some patients remain asymptomatic, and the diagnosis is suggested by a routine ECG

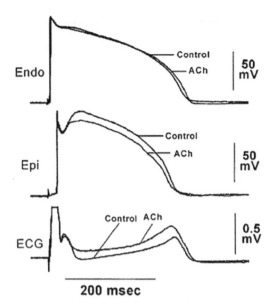

Fig. 2. Acetylcholine (ACh)-induced ST-segment elevation in arterially perfused right ventricular wedge preparation. Transmembrane action potentials from epicardium (Epi) and endocardium (Endo) and an electrocardiogram (ECG) are recorded simultaneously. Superimposed traces are recorded under control conditions and after addition of 3 μmol/L ACh. ACh depresses the action-potential plateau in epicardium but not endocardium and gives rise to the early-repolarization ECG pattern. (*Data from* Yan GX, Antzelevitch C. Cellular basis for the electrocardiographic J wave. Circulation 1996;93:372–9.)

screening showing ST-segment elevation in leads V1 to V3. Many patients report a family history of sudden cardiac death, but the syndrome may also occur sporadically. About 20% of patients complain of atrial fibrillation. Physical examination is usually normal in patients with Brugada syndrome, but it is paramount to exclude other possible cardiac or noncardiac causes for the sudden cardiac arrest or syncope.[40]

The diagnosis of Brugada syndrome requires a combination of (1) ventricular arrhythmias, positive family history, or inducibility at programmed ventricular stimulation; and (2) a type-1 ECG pattern (prominent coved ST-segment elevation displaying J-point amplitude or ST-segment elevation ≥2 mm followed by a negative T wave) in the right precordial leads (V1–V3), either spontaneous or provoked by class-I antiarrhythmic drugs (sodium-channel blockers). Type-2 (≥2 mm J-point elevation, ≥1 mm ST-segment elevation and a saddleback appearance, followed by a positive or biphasic T wave) and type-3 Brugada ECG pattern (either a saddleback or coved appearance, but with an ST-segment elevation <1 mm) are not diagnostic unless administration of sodium-channel blockers unmasks a type-1 Brugada ECG (see **Fig. 3**).[37] According to the consensus on Brugada syndrome, the ECG diagnosis is reached when a type-1 pattern is found in at least 2 right precordial leads (V1–V3); however, a study on 186 Brugada patients established that V3 did not yield diagnostic information in that

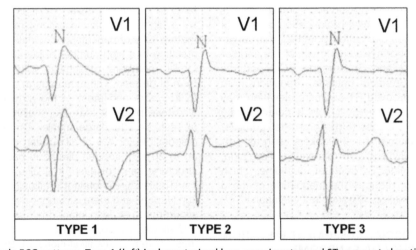

Fig. 3. Brugada ECG patterns. Type 1 (*left*) is characterized by a prominent coved ST-segment elevation displaying J-point amplitude or ST-segment elevation of at least 2 mm followed by a negative T wave. Type 2 (*center*) and type 3 (*right*) are characterized by a J-point elevation of at least 2 mm, a saddleback configuration of the ST segment, and ST-segment elevation of at least 1 mm in type 2 or less than 1 mm in type 3. The type 1 Brugada pattern is the only diagnostic for Brugada syndrome. Conversion from type 2/3 to type 1 Brugada ECG can be observed spontaneously after administration of drugs such as ajmaline and flecainide, or under the influence of factors such as fever or increased parasympathetic stimulation.

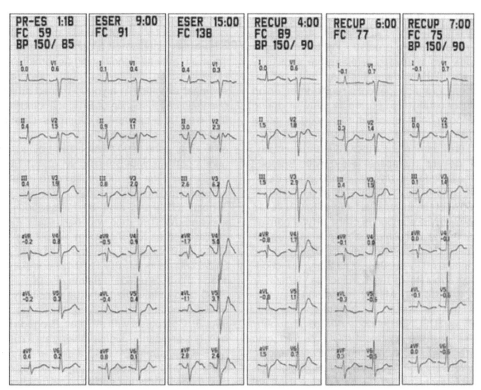

Fig. 4. ECG recorded at preexercise (*PRE-ES*), exercise (*ESER*), and postexercise (*RECUP*) steps in an athlete with Brugada syndrome. Note the distinctive coved-type J-point elevation during recovery as a consequence of the vagal rebound. Sympathetic stimulation aggravates the concomitant intraventricular conduction defect as shown by QRS prolongation from 90 to 130 milliseconds and deeper S waves in inferolateral leads during exercise.

group, and those patients showing a type-1 ECG in only 1 right precordial lead (V1 or V2) presented a clinical profile and arrhythmic risk similar to those of Brugada patients with the same ECG pattern in more than 1 precordial lead.[37,43] In some individuals the degree and morphology of ST-segment elevation may be influenced by lead position, with demonstration of a spontaneous type-1 Brugada ECG only by recording right precordial leads in higher intercostal spaces.[44] A spontaneous type-1 Brugada ECG recorded at standard leads or with higher lead position has the same diagnostic accuracy.[44,45]

GENETIC BASIS OF BRUGADA SYNDROME

Brugada syndrome is an autosomal dominant hereditary condition, and to date 10 genes have been linked to this disease. Mutations of the SCN5A gene leading to a loss of function of the cardiac sodium channel is the most common genotype found in approximately 25% of patients, with almost 300 mutations described.[32,33] Of interest, certain mutations of the SCN5A gene may result in clinical variants of Brugada syndrome characterized by an enhanced risk of sudden death

during sports performance. A single C-terminal aspartic acid insertion (1795insD) has been described to lead to the ECG manifestations of both long-QT and Brugada syndromes: QT-interval prolongation and distinctive right precordial ST-segment elevations.[46] The mutation affects the fast inactivation component of the sodium channel, causing a plateau of persistent sodium current that prolongs the QT interval at slow heart rates. At the same time, 1795insD induces depolarized sodium channels to undergo excessive slow inactivation, which reduces sodium-channel availability primarily at rapid heart rates. This channel dysfunction accounts for a variant of Brugada syndrome whereby the ST-segment elevation atypically occurs during β-adrenergic stimulation. The 1795insD carriers are expected to exhibit right precordial ST-segment elevation and to increase their arrhythmic risk during an enhanced sympathetic drive such as during sports exercise. The threonine at position 1620 in the coding sequence of SCN5A is an important determinant of the temperature sensitivity of the human cardiac sodium channel.[47] This missense mutation (Thr1620Met) causes a temperature-dependent speeding up of the inactivation of the sodium current, which results in the preponderance of the "outward" early repolarization current, ST-segment elevation, and dispersion of repolarization, predisposing to ventricular fibrillation. This increased temperature sensitivity of the Thr1620Met current decay may predispose some Brugada patients to life-threatening arrhythmias either during a febrile state or during an increase in body temperature caused by intensive physical exercise, mostly if performed in increased environmental temperature and humidity.

Other genetic mutations linked with Brugada syndrome include: the glycerol-3-phosphate dehydrogenase 1–like gene (GPD1L) (leading to reduction of 50% of the inward Na^+ current); CACNA1c and β2b-CACNB2b subunits of the L-type cardiac calcium channel (resulting in a combined Brugada syndrome/short-QT syndrome); SCN1B (encoding for β1- and β1b-subunits, auxiliary function-modifying subunits of the cardiac Na^+ channel); KCNE321 (encoding MiRP2, a protein that decreases the potassium I_{to} by interacting with channel Kv4.3); SCN3B (encodes for the β3-subunit of the Na^+ cardiac channel); MOG123 (reducing Na^+ current); and KCNE524 and KCND325 (leading to an increase of the I_{to}). Each of these 9 genes is responsible for less than 1% of reported cases of Brugada syndrome.[48–55]

DIFFERENTIAL DIAGNOSIS BETWEEN RIGHT PRECORDIAL EARLY REPOLARIZATION AND BRUGADA SYNDROME

Early repolarization is usually characterized by an upward displacement of the ST segment in the inferior and lateral precordial leads. A prominent ST-segment elevation in right precordial leads (right precordial early repolarization) is observed in a minority ($\approx$4%) of trained athletes, in whom it is usually considered a benign consequence of intensive athletic conditioning (ie, athlete's heart). However, the finding of right precordial ST-segment elevation in a young trained athlete may raise clinical suspicion of Brugada syndrome and the need for a differential diagnosis. Corrado and colleagues[56] compared the ECG pattern of right precordial early repolarization in trained athletes and in patients with Brugada syndrome to identify possible criteria for differential diagnosis. Amplitude of maximum ST segment was measured at J point (STJ) and after 80 milliseconds (ST80), and an STJ/ST80 ratio was calculated. Despite a similar degree of maximum amplitude of STJ (3.1 ± 0.9 vs 3.2 ± 0.6 mm), athletes had an STJ/ST80 ratio of 0.7 ± 0.13 compared with 1.6 ± 0.3 in Brugada patients ($P<.001$). An STJ/ST80 ratio of less than 1 had a sensitivity of 87% and a specificity of 100% in identifying athletes (Fig. 5). Compared with athletes, Brugada patients had a significantly higher heart rate (75 ± 9 vs 50 ± 8 beats/min; $P<.001$), a shorter QTc interval (0.35 ± 0.04 vs 0.39 ± 0.02 seconds; $P<.001$), and longer QRS duration ($0.11 \pm 0,02$ vs 0.09 ± 0.01 seconds; $P<.001$), and also more often showed an "S1S2S3 pattern" (53% vs 27%; $P = .04$). The sodium-channel blocker test is usually administered to athletes with an incidental finding of a nondiagnostic Brugada type 2 or 3 ECG pattern to help in the differential diagnosis of Brugada syndrome and early repolarization. In a recent study on the predictive value of such a provocative test, the investigators concluded that the prognostic role of the sodium-channel blocker test in

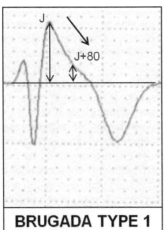
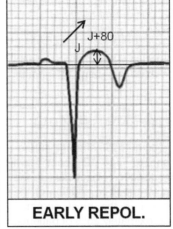

BRUGADA TYPE 1   **EARLY REPOL.**

Fig. 5. Morphologic patterns in a patient with Brugada syndrome (*left*) and a healthy athlete of Afro-Caribbean descent (*right*). The Brugada pattern is characterized by a descending ST segment with an ST_J/ST_{J+80ms} ratio greater than 1. By contrast, the early-repolarization pattern shows an initially ascending ST segment with an ST_J/ST_{J+80ms} ratio less than 1.

individuals with a type-2 or type-3 Brugada ECG varies depending on clinical presentation. In symptomatic patients, the incidence of arrhythmic events during a long-term follow-up was low irrespective of sodium-channel blocker test results, which did not provide additional prognostic and therapeutic value. Therefore, the systematic use of the sodium-channel blocker test for risk stratification of asymptomatic athletes with an incidental nondiagnostic type-2 and type-3 Brugada ECG seems unjustified. On the contrary, in those with a history of either cardiac arrest or unexplained syncope a sodium-channel blocker test is warranted, because it may predict an adverse outcome and contribute to risk stratification and prevention of sudden death.[57]

RISK STRATIFICATION AND SPORTS RECOMMENDATIONS FOR PATIENTS WITH BRUGADA SYNDROME

Large-scale cohort studies on the clinical outcome of patients with Brugada syndrome have consistently demonstrated that symptomatic patients with documented ventricular tachyarrhythmias, cardiac arrest, and/or syncope (after the exclusion of noncardiac causes) have a significantly higher risk of sudden death than do asymptomatic patients. In particular, a recent study on the largest series of Brugada patients (FINGER study) reported an annual sudden death rate of 7.7% among survivors of cardiac arrest, 1.5% among patients with a history of syncope, and 0.5% among asymptomatic individuals.[58] These results were reproduced by the PRELUDE study, which investigated the predictive value of induction of ventricular tachycardia/ventricular fibrillation (VT/VF) by programmed ventricular stimulation, and concluded that VT/VF inducibility is unable to identify high-risk patients, whereas the presence of a spontaneous type-1 ECG, history of syncope, ventricular effective refractory period shorter than 200 milliseconds, and QRS fragmentation seem useful in identifying candidates for prophylactic implantable cardioverter-defibrillators.[59] On the other hand, a recent retrospective study reported that cardiac arrest was the first clinical manifestation in the majority of victims of sudden death from Brugada syndrome, thus suggesting a possible survivor bias in the large-scale registry studies. The independent predicting value of other clinical variables such as male sex, family history of sudden death, inducibility at programmed ventricular stimulation, and a spontaneous type-1 Brugada ECG remains elusive. In addition, the prognostic value and the clinical utility of molecular genetic analysis has not yet been demonstrated.

According to the European and American recommendations, symptomatic patients with Brugada syndrome are currently treated with implantable defibrillator therapy with its inherent limitations in sports practice.[60] Although an increased vagal tone as a consequence of sustained athletic conditioning may enhance the propensity to die suddenly at rest, no data exist that directly relate asymptomatic patients, Brugada-gene carriers without ECG abnormalities, or asymptomatic family members to the risk of participating in sports. For this subgroup of individuals the European recommendations allow all recreational and competitive sports. However, the American recommendations still restrict those in this group to only low-intensity sports to avoid the potential harmful impact of hyperthermia.

INFEROLATERAL EARLY REPOLARIZATION AND THE EARLY REPOLARIZATION SYNDROME

Physiologic early repolarization is characterized by a distinct notch at the J point (J wave) or slur on the downslope of the R wave associated with upsloping ST segment and tall T waves.[61] It has an estimated prevalence of 1% to 2% in healthy young individuals and up to 50% to 80% in highly trained athletes, particularly if male and of Afro-Caribbean descent.[56] As it reflects the physiologic electrical adaptation of the heart to physical exercise, early repolarization has been traditionally considered not only a benign ECG sign but also a marker of good health.[62] However, this perspective has recently been challenged.

Experimental studies first indicated that the presence of a transmural electrical heterogeneity, giving rise to the early-repolarization ECG pattern, may favor malignant arrhythmias under certain conditions (ischemia, electrolytic imbalance, hypothermia, and use of specific drugs).[28] Clinically the association of early repolarization with increased risk for ventricular arrhythmias was first noted for hypothermia.[63] In the last decade there have been several case reports on patients with idiopathic ventricular fibrillation, (ie, ventricular fibrillation in the absence of known heart diseases), showing prominent early repolarization and augmentation of the ST-segment elevation at the J point before the onset of malignant arrhythmias.[13,17,19,21,22] In 2008, Haïssaguerre and colleagues[11] published a seminal case-control multicenter study including 206 cases of idiopathic ventricular fibrillation and 412 control subjects matched for age, sex, race, and level of physical activity. The investigators reported a 31% prevalence of early repolarization in the idiopathic ventricular fibrillation group versus 5% in the control group (P<.001). In 91% of patients early repolarization involved the inferior limb leads (II, III, aVF), whereas it was confined to the lateral leads (I, aVL, V4–V6) in only 9% of cases. The association between early repolarization in the inferior ± lateral leads and idiopathic ventricular fibrillation was termed early repolarization syndrome, and was confirmed by other case-control studies.[9,14,18,64] An increased prevalence of early repolarization was also found among 21 athletes who had been resuscitated from ventricular fibrillation or who suffered sudden death without evidence of structural heart disease.[10] Finally, inferolateral early repolarization was recognized as a risk factor for cardiovascular death in the general population.[12,16,20,65] A plausible explanation is that subjects with J waves are more prone to develop ventricular fibrillation when exposed to additional proarrhythmic factors, particularly myocardial ischemia.[66]

Laboratory examinations and clinical observations (ie, response to isoproterenol infusion or β-blocker administration, higher incidence of arrhythmic events during sleep, high prevalence of family history of sudden death, increase in the amplitude of J-point elevation before the arrhythmic event, phase-2 reentry mechanism) suggest that Brugada syndrome and early repolarization syndrome share the same electrophysiologic substrate. Although the 2 syndromes differ with respect to the magnitude (more pronounced in Brugada syndrome than in early repolarization syndrome) and lead location (right precordial leads in the former, inferolateral leads in the latter) of the J waves, they can be considered to represent 2 phenotypic expressions of the same physiopathologic mechanism (J-wave syndromes).[24]

DIFFERENTIAL DIAGNOSIS BETWEEN BENIGN AND MALIGNANT INFEROLATERAL EARLY REPOLARIZATION
Location of ECG Leads

Based on the aforementioned studies, 3 early repolarization variants according to lead location have been identified[23]:

- Type 1: Early repolarization predominantly in the lateral precordial leads (V4–V6). This pattern is rarely seen in cases of idiopathic ventricular fibrillation, whereas it is highly prevalent among healthy young adults and athletes.
- Type 2: Early repolarization in the inferior or inferolateral leads. This pattern is less common in the general population, whereas

it is observed in approximately 50% of cases of idiopathic ventricular fibrillation. Early repolarization in the inferior leads is also associated with an increased risk of cardiovascular death from any cause.
- Type 3: Early repolarization in both the right precordial leads and inferolateral leads. This pattern is the rarest and carries the highest risk of malignant ventricular arrhythmias.

J-Wave Amplitude

In the study by Haïssaguerre and colleagues,[11] patients with idiopathic ventricular fibrillation had significantly greater amplitude of J-point elevation than controls, and subjects with extreme J-point elevation (>0.5 mV) carried the highest risk. A nonsignificant trend between the degree of J-point elevation and the risk for idiopathic ventricular fibrillation was also reported by Rosso and colleagues.[18] Finally, in the general population the probability of death from cardiac causes in subjects with early repolarization is higher if J-point elevation is at least 0.2 mV.[65]

ST-Segment Configuration

Tikannen and colleagues[67] reanalyzed their original study population, and found that an upsloping ST segment is very common among young athletes and has no adverse clinical implications. By contrast, the combination of J-point elevation or slurred R waves with a horizontal/descending ST segment is strongly associated with an increased risk of cardiovascular death at follow-up. Rosso and colleagues[68] performed the same analysis in their subjects with early repolarization syndrome, and found that a horizontal/descending ST segment improved the distinction between patients with idiopathic ventricular fibrillation and healthy controls. In particular, they observed that only 15% of athletes and 25% of adult controls with early repolarization showed a horizontal/descending ST segment compared with approximately 70% of patients with the early repolarization syndrome. In this study, the pattern of horizontal/descending ST segment yielded an odds ratio of 13.8 for having idiopathic ventricular fibrillation. Finally, Cappato and colleagues[10] found the presence of ST-segment elevation to be not statistically different in athletes with idiopathic ventricular fibrillation when compared with controls. However, the presence of J wave and/or QRS slurring without ST-segment elevation was more frequently observed in victims of cardiac arrest or sudden death than in control athletes (38.1% vs 15.6%, P = .04), particularly in the inferior leads (23.8% vs 2.5%, P = .001)[10] (Fig. 6).

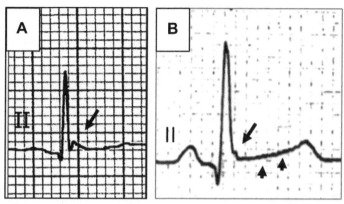

Fig. 6. Early-repolarization patterns in the inferior limb L2 in a 47-year-old sedentary patient with idiopathic ventricular fibrillation (*A*) and an 18-year-old healthy athlete (*B*). The patient exhibited a J wave (*arrow*) followed by a horizontal ST segment, whereas the athlete showed an ascending ST segment (*upward arrows*).

Race

The association between early repolarization and sudden death has been established only in Caucasian or Asian subjects. In studies including individuals of Afro-Caribbean descent, the association between early repolarization and sudden cardiac death did not reach statistical significance.[11,16,69]

IMPLICATIONS FOR SCREENING OF ATHLETES

The incidental finding of early repolarization in the ECG of an apparently healthy athlete may raise the concern of an underlying arrhythmic substrate at risk for sudden death during sports activity. However, to put the studies on the association between idiopathic ventricular fibrillation and early repolarization into clinical perspective, it must be kept in mind that in highly trained athletes the former is an extremely rare condition and the latter is the rule. According to the Bayes formula, it has been calculated that finding a J wave and/or QRS slurring in an athlete increases the probability of experiencing idiopathic ventricular fibrillation from 2 in 1,000,000 to 3.5 in 1,000,000.[10] Even the "malignant" pattern of J waves without ST-segment elevation in the inferior leads is found in 3% to 4% of healthy athletes and carries an estimated odds for developing idiopathic ventricular fibrillation of only 1 in 30,000.[10,68,70]

Given these considerations, in asymptomatic athletes early repolarization should still be considered a physiologic ECG pattern reflecting cardiac adaptation to exercise, and this is particularly true for individuals of Afro-Caribbean descent.[56,66,71] However, in athletes with a family history of unexplained sudden death or a personal history of syncope or cardiac arrest with no evidence of structural heart disease, the ECG pattern of early repolarization should raise the suspicion of an idiopathic ventricular fibrillation, especially if it involves the inferior limb leads, and if the J-point is markedly elevated and is associated with a flat or descending ST segment.[56,68]

REFERENCES

1. Thiene G, Basso C. Sudden coronary death—not always atherosclerotic. Heart 2010;96:1084–5.
2. Corrado D, Basso C, Thiene G. Sudden cardiac death in young people with apparently normal heart. Cardiovasc Res 2001;50:399–408.
3. Tester DJ, Ackerman MJ. The role of molecular autopsy in unexplained sudden cardiac death. Curr Opin Cardiol 2006;21:166–72.
4. Basso C, Carturan E, Pilichou K, et al. Sudden cardiac death with normal heart: molecular autopsy. Cardiovasc Pathol 2010;19:321–5.
5. Chugh SS, Kelly KL, Titus JL. Sudden cardiac death with apparently normal heart. Circulation 2000;102:649–54.
6. Basso C, Calabrese F, Corrado D, et al. Postmortem diagnosis in sudden cardiac death victims: macroscopic, microscopic and molecular findings. Cardiovasc Res 2001;50:290–300.
7. Brugada J, Brugada R, Brugada P. Right bundle-branch block and ST-segment elevation in leads V1 through V3: a marker for sudden death in patients without demonstrable structural heart disease. Circulation 1998;97:457–60.
8. Brugada P, Brugada J. Right bundle branch block, persistent ST-segment elevation and sudden cardiac death: a distinct clinical and electrocardiographic syndrome. A multicenter report. J Am Coll Cardiol 1992;20:1391–6.

9. Abe A, Ikeda T, Tsukada T, et al. Circadian variation of late potentials in idiopathic ventricular fibrillation associated with J waves: insights into alternative pathophysiology and risk stratification. Heart Rhythm 2010;7:675–82.

10. Cappato R, Furlanello F, Giovinazzo V, et al. J wave, QRS slurring, and ST elevation in athletes with cardiac arrest in the absence of heart disease: marker of risk or innocent bystander? Circ Arrhythm Electrophysiol 2010;3:305–11.

11. Haïssaguerre M, Derval N, Sacher F, et al. Sudden cardiac arrest associated with early repolarization. N Engl J Med 2008;358:2016–23.

12. Haruta D, Matsuo K, Tsuneto A, et al. Incidence and prognostic value of early repolarization pattern in the 12-lead electrocardiogram. Circulation 2011;123: 2931–7.

13. Komiya N, Imanishi R, Kawano H, et al. Ventricular fibrillation in a patient with prominent j wave in the inferior and lateral electrocardiographic leads after gastrostomy. Pacing Clin Electrophysiol 2006;29: 1022–4.

14. Merchant FM, Noseworthy PA, Weiner RB, et al. Ability of terminal QRS notching to distinguish benign from malignant electrocardiographic forms of early repolarization. Am J Cardiol 2009;104: 1402–6.

15. Nam GB, Kim YH, Antzelevitch C. Augmentation of J waves and electrical storms in patients with early repolarization. N Engl J Med 2008;358: 2078–9.

16. Olson KA, Viera AJ, Soliman EZ, et al. Long-term prognosis associated with J-point elevation in a large middle-aged biracial cohort: the ARIC study. Eur Heart J 2011;32:3098–106.

17. Riera AR, Ferreira C, Schapachnik E, et al. Brugada syndrome with atypical ECG: downsloping ST-segment elevation in inferior leads. J Electrocardiol 2004;37:101–4.

18. Rosso R, Kogan E, Belhassen B, et al. J-point elevation in survivors of primary ventricular fibrillation and matched control subjects: incidence and clinical significance. J Am Coll Cardiol 2008;52:1231–8.

19. Sahara M, Sagara K, Yamashita T, et al. J wave and ST-segment elevation in the inferior leads: a latent type of variant Brugada syndrome? Jpn Heart J 2002;43:55–60.

20. Sinner MF, Reinhard W, Muller M, et al. Association of early repolarization pattern on ECG with risk of cardiac and all-cause mortality: a population-based prospective cohort study (MONICA/KORA). PLoS Med 2010;7:e1000314.

21. Sugao M, Fujiki A, Nishida K, et al. Repolarization dynamics in patients with idiopathic ventricular fibrillation: pharmacological therapy with bepridil and disopyramide. J Cardiovasc Pharmacol 2005;45: 545–9.

22. Tsunoda Y, Takeishi Y, Nozaki N, et al. Presence of intermittent J waves in multiple leads in relation to episode of atrial and ventricular fibrillation. J Electrocardiol 2004;37:311–4.

23. Antzelevitch C, Yan GX. J wave syndromes. Heart Rhythm 2010;7:549–58.

24. Antzelevitch C, Yan GX, Viskin S. Rationale for the use of the terms J-wave syndromes and early repolarization. J Am Coll Cardiol 2011;57:1587–90.

25. Corrado D, McKenna WJ. Appropriate interpretation of the athlete's electrocardiogram saves lives as well as money. Eur Heart J 2007;28:1920–2.

26. Yan GX, Antzelevitch C. Cellular basis for the electrocardiographic J wave. Circulation 1996;93: 372–9.

27. Yan GX, Antzelevitch C. Cellular basis for the Brugada syndrome and other mechanisms of arrhythmogenesis associated with ST-segment elevation. Circulation 1999;100:1660–6.

28. Gussak I, Antzelevitch C. Early repolarization syndrome: clinical characteristics and possible cellular and ionic mechanisms. J Electrocardiol 2000;33: 299–309.

29. Yan GX, Lankipalli RS, Burke JF, et al. Ventricular repolarization components on the electrocardiogram: cellular basis and clinical significance. J Am Coll Cardiol 2003;42:401–9.

30. Litovsky SH, Antzelevitch C. Differences in the electrophysiological response of canine ventricular subendocardium and subepicardium to acetylcholine and isoproterenol. A direct effect of acetylcholine in ventricular myocardium. Circ Res 1990;67: 615–27.

31. Bianco M, Bria S, Gianfelici A, et al. Does early repolarization in the athlete have analogies with the Brugada syndrome? Eur Heart J 2001;22:504–10.

32. Kapplinger JD, Tester DJ, Alders M, et al. An international compendium of mutations in the SCN5A-encoded cardiac sodium channel in patients referred for Brugada syndrome genetic testing. Heart Rhythm 2010;7:33–46.

33. Chen Q, Kirsch GE, Zhang D, et al. Genetic basis and molecular mechanism for idiopathic ventricular fibrillation. Nature 1998;392:293–6.

34. Antzelevitch C. Brugada syndrome. Pacing Clin Electrophysiol 2006;29:1130–59.

35. Hong K, Brugada J, Oliva A, et al. Value of electrocardiographic parameters and ajmaline test in the diagnosis of Brugada syndrome caused by SCN5A mutations. Circulation 2004;110:3023–7.

36. Meregalli PG, Ruijter JM, Hofman N, et al. Diagnostic value of flecainide testing in unmasking SCN5A-related Brugada syndrome. J Cardiovasc Electrophysiol 2006;17:857–64.

37. Antzelevitch C, Brugada P, Borggrefe M, et al. Brugada syndrome: report of the second consensus conference: endorsed by the Heart Rhythm Society

and the European Heart Rhythm Association. Circulation 2005;111:659–70.

38. Donohue D, Tehrani F, Jamehdor R, et al. The prevalence of Brugada ECG in adult patients in a large university hospital in the western United States. Am Heart Hosp J 2008;6:48–50.

39. Miyasaka Y, Tsuji H, Yamada K, et al. Prevalence and mortality of the Brugada-type electrocardiogram in one city in Japan. J Am Coll Cardiol 2001; 38:771–4.

40. Berne P, Brugada J. Brugada syndrome 2012. Circ J 2012;76:1563–71.

41. Amin AS, Meregalli PG, Bardai A, et al. Fever increases the risk for cardiac arrest in the Brugada syndrome. Ann Intern Med 2008;149:216–8.

42. Postema PG, Wolpert C, Amin AS, et al. Drugs and Brugada syndrome patients: review of the literature, recommendations, and an up-to-date website (www.brugadadrugs.org). Heart Rhythm 2009;6: 1335–41.

43. Richter S, Sarkozy A, Paparella G, et al. Number of electrocardiogram leads displaying the diagnostic coved-type pattern in Brugada syndrome: a diagnostic consensus criterion to be revised. Eur Heart J 2010;31:1357–64.

44. Shimeno K, Takagi M, Maeda K, et al. Usefulness of multichannel Holter ECG recording in the third intercostal space for detecting type 1 Brugada ECG: comparison with repeated 12-lead ECGs. J Cardiovasc Electrophysiol 2009;20:1026–31.

45. Miyamoto K, Yokokawa M, Tanaka K, et al. Diagnostic and prognostic value of a type 1 Brugada electrocardiogram at higher (third or second) V1 to V2 recording in men with Brugada syndrome. Am J Cardiol 2007;99:53–7.

46. Bezzina C, Veldkamp MW, van Den Berg MP, et al. A single Na(+) channel mutation causing both long-QT and Brugada syndromes. Circ Res 1999; 85:1206–13.

47. Dumaine R, Towbin JA, Brugada P, et al. Ionic mechanisms responsible for the electrocardiographic phenotype of the Brugada syndrome are temperature dependent. Circ Res 1999;85:803–9.

48. London B, Michalec M, Mehdi H, et al. Mutation in glycerol-3-phosphate dehydrogenase 1 like gene (GPD1-L) decreases cardiac Na+ current and causes inherited arrhythmias. Circulation 2007;116: 2260–8.

49. Antzelevitch C, Pollevick GD, Cordeiro JM, et al. Loss-of-function mutations in the cardiac calcium channel underlie a new clinical entity characterized by ST-segment elevation, short QT intervals, and sudden cardiac death. Circulation 2007;115: 442–9.

50. Watanabe H, Koopmann TT, Le Scouarnec S, et al. Sodium channel beta1 subunit mutations associated with Brugada syndrome and cardiac conduction disease in humans. J Clin Invest 2008;118:2260–8.

51. Delpon E, Cordeiro JM, Nunez L, et al. Functional effects of KCNE3 mutation and its role in the development of Brugada syndrome. Circ Arrhythm Electrophysiol 2008;1:209–18.

52. Hu D, Barajas-Martinez H, Burashnikov E, et al. A mutation in the beta 3 subunit of the cardiac sodium channel associated with Brugada ECG phenotype. Circ Cardiovasc Genet 2009;2:270–8.

53. Kattygnarath D, Maugenre S, Neyroud N, et al. MOG1: a new susceptibility gene for Brugada syndrome. Circ Cardiovasc Genet 2011;4:261–8.

54. Ohno S, Zankov DP, Ding WG, et al. KCNE5 (KCNE1L) variants are novel modulators of Brugada syndrome and idiopathic ventricular fibrillation. Circ Arrhythm Electrophysiol 2011;4:352–61.

55. Giudicessi JR, Ye D, Tester DJ, et al. Transient outward current (I(to)) gain-of-function mutations in the KCND3-encoded Kv4.3 potassium channel and Brugada syndrome. Heart Rhythm 2011;8:1024–32.

56. Corrado D, Pelliccia A, Heidbuchel H, et al. Recommendations for interpretation of 12-lead electrocardiogram in the athlete. Eur Heart J 2010;31:243–59.

57. Zorzi A, Migliore F, Marras E, et al. Should all individuals with a nondiagnostic Brugada-electrocardiogram undergo sodium-channel blocker test? Heart Rhythm 2012;9:909–16.

58. Probst V, Veltmann C, Eckardt L, et al. Long-term prognosis of patients diagnosed with Brugada syndrome: results from the FINGER Brugada Syndrome Registry. Circulation 2010;121:635–43.

59. Priori SG, Gasparini M, Napolitano C, et al. Risk stratification in Brugada syndrome: results of the PRELUDE (PRogrammed ELectrical stimUlation preDictive valuE) registry. J Am Coll Cardiol 2012; 59:37–45.

60. Pelliccia A, Zipes DP, Maron BJ. Bethesda Conference #36 and the European Society of Cardiology Consensus Recommendations revisited a comparison of U.S. and European criteria for eligibility and disqualification of competitive athletes with cardiovascular abnormalities. J Am Coll Cardiol 2008;52: 1990–6.

61. Wasserburger RH, Alt WJ. The normal RS-T segment elevation variant. Am J Cardiol 1961;8:184–92.

62. Klatsky AL, Oehm R, Cooper RA, et al. The early repolarization normal variant electrocardiogram: correlates and consequences. Am J Med 2003; 115:171–7.

63. Osborn JJ. Experimental hypothermia; respiratory and blood pH changes in relation to cardiac function. Am J Physiol 1953;175:389–98.

64. Nam GB, Ko KH, Kim J, et al. Mode of onset of ventricular fibrillation in patients with early repolarization pattern vs. Brugada syndrome. Eur Heart J 2010;31:330–9.

65. Tikkanen JT, Anttonen O, Junttila MJ, et al. Long-term outcome associated with early repolarization on electrocardiography. N Engl J Med 2009;361: 2529–37.

66. Rosso R, Adler A, Halkin A, et al. Risk of sudden death among young individuals with J waves and early repolarization: putting the evidence into perspective. Heart Rhythm 2011;8:923–9.

67. Tikkanen JT, Junttila MJ, Anttonen O, et al. Early repolarization: electrocardiographic phenotypes associated with favorable long-term outcome. Circulation 2011;123:2666–73.

68. Rosso R, Glikson E, Belhassen B, et al. Distinguishing "benign" from "malignant early repolarization": the value of the ST-segment morphology. Heart Rhythm 2012;9:225–9.

69. Perez MV, Uberoi A, Jain NA, et al. The prognostic value of early repolarization with ST-segment elevation in African Americans. Heart Rhythm 2012;9:558–65.

70. Noseworthy PA, Tikkanen JT, Porthan K, et al. The early repolarization pattern in the general population: clinical correlates and heritability. J Am Coll Cardiol 2011;57:2284–9.

71. Papadakis M, Carre F, Kervio G, et al. The prevalence, distribution, and clinical outcomes of electrocardiographic repolarization patterns in male athletes of African/Afro-Caribbean origin. Eur Heart J 2011;32:2304–13.

Syncope in the Athlete

Yousef H. Bader, MD, Mark S. Link, MD*

KEYWORDS

- Athlete • Syncope • Hypertrophic cardiomyopathy
- Arrhythmogenic right ventricular cardiomyopathy • Brugada syndrome • Long QT syndrome
- Commotio cordis

KEY POINTS

- Syncope during sports may be secondary to nonsustained ventricular arrhythmias and thus a precursor of sudden cardiac death; however, not all syncope is life threatening.
- When syncope occurs, it is important to quickly identify the cause and begin the proper steps to manage these conditions; the history is of paramount importance and guides further work-up and management.
- In most cases, syncope that occurs during exercise is concerning, whereas syncope after exertion is usually benign.
- Neurally mediated syncope and postexercise collapse usually occur after cessation of exercise and are generally benign conditions.
- Persistent delirium after collapse is life threatening and generally caused by hyperthermia or hyponatremia.

Syncope in an athlete during intense exercise is unexpected and concerning. This rare occurrence is ominous because syncope may be secondary to nonsustained ventricular arrhythmias and thus a precursor of sudden cardiac death (SCD). However, the causes of syncope in the athlete range from benign problems to fatal ventricular arrhythmias. When such an event occurs, it is important to quickly identify the cause and begin the proper steps to manage the condition. In most cases, syncope that occurs during exercise is concerning, whereas syncope after exertion is usually benign. Neurally mediated syncope (NMS) and postexertion collapse usually occur after cessation of exercise and are generally benign conditions. The history is paramount in the differential diagnosis of syncope and should have 3 parts: before the event, during syncope, and after awakening.[1–3]

NONARRHYTHMIC CAUSES OF SYNCOPE

Neurally Mediated Syncope

As in nonathletes, the most common cause of syncope in athletes is NMS.[4] In athletes, NMS occurs not during exertion but after activity, such as during a time-out or huddle or at the end of a race.[5–9] Specific triggers such as blood draws and prolonged standing are common; individuals are usually in an upright posture. Classic prodromal symptoms include lightheadedness, warmth, nausea, tunnel vision, and palpitations. Individuals tend to slump to the ground rather than drop suddenly. As such, injury is unusual because they are not fully unconscious until after they are on the ground. Syncope is brief (5–30 seconds) and patients awake nauseous and exhausted. In many, the exhaustion is so profound that they do not feel normal until they have slept.

Disclosures: No conflicts of interest to declare.
The Cardiac Arrhythmia Center, Department of Medicine, Tufts Medical Center, 800 Washington Street, Boston, MA 02111, USA
* Corresponding author. Tufts Medical Center, Box #197, 800 Washington Street, Boston, MA 02111.
E-mail address: mlink@tuftsmedicalcenter.org

The pathophysiologic mechanisms of NMS are incompletely understood. Some studies suggest that, in athletes, blood pressure control is impaired as a result of depressed carotid baroreflex sensitivity.[6] Endurance athletes have more compliant, distensible ventricles associated with a chronic volume load during training, and therefore, compared with nonathletes, have a steeper slope of the Frank-Starling curve relating left ventricular (LV) filling pressure to stroke volume. The increase in chamber compliance and steep Frank-Starling curve, facilitating the delivery of a large volume of blood to the exercising muscle, is beneficial to the performing athlete.[10] However, it may be a disadvantage during orthostasis, resulting in a large decrease in stroke volume when filling pressure is reduced.[5]

Another possibility is that a rapid decrease in venous return to the heart after exertion causes more vigorous ventricular contraction that activates mechanoreceptors causing increased afferent neural output. This sudden surge of neural input to the brainstem is thought to produce bradycardia and peripheral vascular dilatation.[6,7]

Postexertion Collapse

Syncope immediately after exercise, also known as postexertion collapse, accounts for a significant percentage of syncope in the athlete.[11] In a study of marathon runners seeking medical attention (2.5%) after an event, 70% were caused by postexertion collapse.[12] This syndrome occurs after profound exertion and usually occurs shortly after finishing a competitive race. Prodromal symptoms are fatigue and pallor. As in NMS, patients slump to the ground protecting themselves from severe injury with outstretched arms. Consciousness is often not completely lost. Individuals may remain symptomatic with fatigue for a long period and frequently require medical attention, but confusion and delirium are unusual and suggest a more severe disorder.[11]

Postexertion collapse was previously thought to be caused by dehydration and hyperthermia. However, it seems that postexertion collapse is caused by pooling of blood in the lower extremities leading to postural hypotension. A study by Holtzhausen and colleagues[13] followed 31 marathon runners and found that there was no relationship between postexertion syncope and body temperature or dehydration. Exercise-associated collapse is thought to be, in part, caused by cardiac remodeling. Athletes' hearts have mild dilatation of the left ventricle and mild to moderate increase in LV wall thickness leading to an increased cardiac output. In the setting of exercise, the lower extremity muscles require an increase in blood flow, which is achieved by decreasing peripheral vascular resistance. The contracting skeletal muscle during exercise ensures adequate return of blood to the heart and maintenance of a constant preload. At the end of exercise, when peripheral resistance is still low, skeletal muscle is no longer contracting. The resultant loss of venous return of blood leads to a large volume of blood pooling in the lower extremities and syncope. Although uncomfortable for the athlete, postexertion collapse is a benign condition and is differentiated from other causes of syncope by the absence of neurologic, biochemical, and thermal abnormalities.

Hyperthermia and Hyponatremia

Collapse of the athlete with changes in temperature or neurologic status after exercise are concerning and are likely to be secondary to hyperthermia or hyponatremia. These conditions are more likely during heat and prolonged training or competition. Prodromal symptoms include confusion and delirium, and staggering during competition. Unlike postexertion collapse, collapse can occur any time during the race. These individuals may slump to the ground, preventing serious trauma, or collapse more suddenly. As in postexertion collapse, full loss of consciousness may not occur. After collapse, individuals continue to have symptoms of confusion and even delirium, and these persist until the hyperthermia or hyponatremia are reversed. These individuals require immediate medical attention to prevent long-term adverse effects and even death.[11,14]

Hyperthermia leading to syncope, or heat syncope, is a part of a spectrum called heat illness.[15] It is thought to be caused by a decrease in cardiac output from postural hypotension secondary to prolonged dehydration. The diagnosis of heat syncope is based on the presence of a core temperature greater than or equal to 40°C and central nervous system dysfunction.[15–17] Heat can also cause syncope in athletes by other mechanisms. Excessive sweating in athletes because of heat leads to a loss of sodium in sweat resulting in hyponatremia. It is also thought that athletes involved in sports with prolonged exercise experience hyponatremia caused by abnormal fluid retention, which is not related to serum vasopressin levels. Athletes often rehydrate with water, leading to further reductions in serum sodium levels, which manifests clinically as altered mental status and occasionally syncope.[18]

Seizures

Although not technically syncope, seizures are important because they are frequently in the differential diagnosis. In contrast with syncope, which is defined as loss of consciousness with loss of muscle tone, seizure is loss of consciousness with increased muscle tone. Both seizure and cerebral hypoperfusion cause abnormal motor movements. Seizures cause loss of consciousness and motor disorders simultaneously, whereas cerebral hypoperfusion causes loss of consciousness followed by myoclonus 5 to 10 seconds later. Prodromal symptoms include specific auras. Injury is common and seizures can be prolonged. The postictal state is of global confusion with slow clearing of sensorium.

CARDIAC CAUSES OF SYNCOPE

Cardiac causes of syncope can be either structural or a primary arrhythmic condition and account for approximately 1% of syncope in the athlete.[19] In these causes of syncope, there is often little or no prodrome. If symptoms occur before syncope, they are brief and consist largely of lightheadedness and visual changes (graying of vision). With cardiac causes of syncope, the individual is unconscious before hitting the ground, thus injury is common. Episodes are brief and generally less than 15 seconds. Although there is initial confusion about how the athlete fell to the ground, they generally feel well after syncope, and frequently do not seek medical attention.

Bradyarrhythmias

Most endurance athletes have resting sinus bradycardia that is attributed to high vagal tone. However, trained athletes had longer sinus cycle length, sinus node recovery time, and AV nodal Wenckebach that persisted despite the use of atropine and propranolol, suggesting that these changes were caused by changes in the intrinsic physiology of the SA and AV nodes in addition to a high vagal tone.[20] First-degree atrioventricular block and Wenckebach are common findings in athletes and have no implications in asymptomatic individuals. Mobitz type II and complete heart block are uncommon in athletes and warrant further investigation and usually intervention. Symptoms are likely to occur during exercise because of the athlete's inability to mount an appropriate heart rate response, leading to a decreased cardiac output during activity. Athletes with congenital complete heart block may be asymptomatic if they have an adequate junctional escape rhythm. If they are symptomatic and have ventricular ectopy, a ventricular escape, or any structural abnormality, then they require definitive treatment.

Tachyarrhythmias

Tachyarrhythmias causing syncope in the athlete are more ominous than bradyarrhythmias. These tachyarrhythmias can either be caused by primary arrhythmias or underlying conditions resulting in an arrhythmia. Most cases of sudden cardiac death in athletes are attributed to underlying cardiovascular conditions such as hypertrophic cardiomyopathy (HCM), arrhythmogenic right ventricular cardiomyopathy (ARVC), and congenital coronary anomalies.

Hypertrophic Cardiomyopathy

HCM is the most common cause of SCD in athletes, accounting for nearly 45% of SCD. The athlete's heart may undergo certain structural changes that are adaptive in an athlete but would otherwise be pathologic in a nonathletic individual. Evidence of cardiac remodeling secondary to training is seen in approximately 50% of athletes. This evidence includes increases in wall thickness and cavity size. Increases in LV wall thickness vary depending on the type of exercise but, on average, there is about a 10% to 20% increase.[21] This mild cardiac hypertrophy can make it difficult to distinguish between normal physiologic changes and HCM.

Athletes with HCM are at risk of syncope during exercise by 2 mechanisms: LV outflow tract obstruction and arrhythmias. Outflow tract gradients typically increase with exercise and, in some individuals, this gradient becomes high enough to impede forward blood flow, causing exertional syncope. Patients with HCM are also at risk of SCD caused by ventricular arrhythmias, which are often the first clinical presentation of HCM. It is not clear whether the increased risk of SCD in HCM is caused by acute temporal changes of exertion or by chronic remodeling caused by high-intensity athletics. Patients with HCM with a family history of SCD, unexplained syncope, multiple repetitive episodes of nonsustained ventricular tachycardia (VT), and massive LV hypertrophy (LVH) greater than 30 mm are at highest risk of ventricular arrhythmias and SCD.[22]

ARVC

ARVC is responsible for 11% of SCD overall and 22% of SCD in athletes worldwide.[23] In the United States, ARVC is responsible for 4% of SCD in athletes.[24] ARVC is a genetic disorder leading to defects in desmosomal proteins, which in turn leads to fibrofatty replacement of myocardium. This disease affects the right ventricle in about 95% of cases and, in about 50% of those cases, there is also LV involvement. Patients develop VTs originating from the right ventricle, which appear as left bundle branch block morphology on an electrocardiogram (ECG). Right ventricular outflow tract (RVOT) tachycardia is the most common VT seen in these patients and differentiation from idiopathic RVOT VT is occasionally difficult. Task force criteria for ARVC have recently been updated.[25] The most common ECG finding in ARVC is T-wave inversions in leads V1 to V3; 50% of patients also have an epsilon wave, a terminal notch seen at the end of the QRS complex resulting from post-excitation of cardiac myocytes in the right ventricle.

Coronary Anomalies

Coronary anomalies are the second most common cause of athletic SCD in the United States, accounting for approximately 17%.[26] The most common coronary anomaly is a left anomalous coronary artery arising from the right coronary sinus. A slitlike orifice of the coronary ostium, the presence of an intramural segment within the aortic wall, and a large territory of myocardium supplied by the anomalous coronary are all high-risk features.[27] Athletes with anomalous coronaries may be asymptomatic but, when syncope occurs, it is often a harbinger of SCD.[28]

Commotio Cordis

Commotio cordis is responsible for up to 20% of sudden cardiac deaths in athletes in the United States and is seen in high-impact sports such as baseball, hockey, and boxing.[26,29,30] Nonsustained arrhythmias causing syncope may also be secondary to chest wall impact. Several important variables, including timing, site and velocity of impact, and shape and hardness of impact object, must be met in order for arrhythmias to occur.[31–33] Susceptibility to commotio cordis is present in the young[29] and is possibly also genetically determined.[34]

Long QT Syndrome

The long QT syndrome (LQTS) is a group of genetically inherited disorders affecting cardiac ion channels, which result in prolonged ventricular repolarization and may lead to polymorphic VT. Although there are currently 13 different types of LQTS, LQT types 1, 2, and 3 account for 75% of inherited syndromes.[35] Athletes with a LQTS may be asymptomatic or may have sudden-onset palpitations, presyncope, syncope, or even sudden cardiac death caused by the development of torsades de pointes.[36] It is estimated that long QT causes 0.5% to 8% of SCD in athletes.[37]

Brugada Syndrome

Brugada syndrome may be acquired, but most commonly is an autosomal dominant condition caused by a loss-of-function mutation in the SCN5A gene, and it is most prevalent in southeast Asia. Athletes with Brugada syndrome most commonly present with palpitations or unexplained syncope and, less frequently, with ventricular fibrillation and sudden cardiac death. Unlike many other arrhythmic conditions, ventricular arrhythmias in patients with Brugada are enhanced by a higher vagal tone and thus SCD most frequently occurs during sleep. Arrhythmias in Brugada are also induced by hyperthermia.[38] It is conceivable that athletes with Brugada are more likely to have ventricular arrhythmias than nonathletic Brugada patients, by 2 mechanisms: during exercise, they may have an increase in temperature, inducing ventricular arrhythmias; and arrhythmias may result from their higher vagal tone from training.[38]

RVOT VT

RVOT VT is the most common idiopathic VT in athletes. The principle mechanism of RVOT VT is intracellular calcium overload. During exercise, cyclic adenosine monophosphate levels increase, leading to an increase in intracellular calcium, which in turn, by a mechanism of triggered activity, leads to VT.[39] Some patients have nonsustained repetitive monomorphic VT, whereas others have paroxysmal exercise-induced sustained RVOT VT, which more commonly affects athletes.[40] RVOT VT is usually diagnosed between the third and fifth decades of life. It most frequently occurs during emotional stress or exercise, and athletes usually present with palpitations, presyncope, infrequently syncope, and very rarely, sudden cardiac death.

Catecholaminergic Polymorphic VT

Catecholaminergic polymorphic VT (CPVT) is a genetic disease that is characterized by cardiac electrical instability caused by activation of the sympathetic nervous system. It is most commonly inherited in an autosomal dominant pattern, resulting in mutations in the RYR2 gene; recessive inheritance is caused by mutations in the CASQ2 gene.[41,42] These mutations lead to intracellular calcium loading, which increases the risk of SCD. Because of its inheritance pattern, the mean age of onset is between 7 and 9 years. Athletes with this condition have episodic palpitations, dizziness, or syncope, which most often occur with acute emotion or with exercise. Eighty percent of athletes with this disease have recurrent syncope and 30% have sudden cardiac death.[43] The ECG in patients with CPVT is commonly normal. Syncope is common before the occurrence of SCD.

DIAGNOSIS AND MANAGEMENT
Initial Work-up

The history accounts for most of the work-up of syncope (**Fig. 1**). The history of the event should be broken up into symptoms before (including situational factors and prodromal symptoms), during (including injury, length of episode, motor movements), and after the event (**Table 1**).

Before syncope
Before the event, both situational factors and symptoms should be examined. Situational factors include posture and exertion. NMS generally occurs during standing. A general rule is that syncope occurring during exertion is ominous, whereas syncope occurring immediately after exercise is often benign. Syncope during exertion is more typical of HCM, ARVC, CPVT, and anomalous coronary arteries. Postexertion collapse and hyponatremia/hyperthermia generally occur after or during longer competitive events.

Patients with NMS typically have a short (5–30 seconds) prodrome during which they develop symptoms of warmth, sweating, nausea, dizziness, and change in vision with a gradual loss of consciousness. Athletes with postexertion collapse also have a short prodrome of feeling dizzy and lightheaded, and they gradually also lose consciousness, usually having enough time to protect themselves from the fall.

During syncope
During the event, characteristics such as time course, motor activity, and (perhaps most importantly) injury are important because of the prodrome and the gradual loss of consciousness. Patients with NMS usually do not hurt themselves because they have time to block their fall. The same is generally true of postexertion collapse and hyperthermia/hyponatremia. In any of these three, collapse without complete loss of consciousness is possible. In contrast, injury is common in cardiac causes of syncope and seizures because athletes are unconscious at the time of collapse and thus do not break their falls. In addition, many patients with cardiac syncope have no prodrome of symptoms. Myoclonus

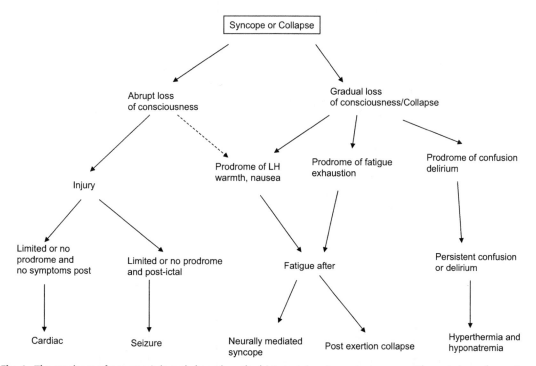

Fig. 1. The work-up of syncope is largely based on the history. Injury is most common with acute loss of consciousness from cardiac causes, syncope, and so on. However, injury can occasionally be seen with other causes of collapse. After the syncope/collapse, patients with cardiac causes frequently return to normal immediately, whereas those with seizures, neurally mediated syncope, postexertion collapse, and hyperthermia/hyponatremia have persistent symptoms. If there is persistent delirium, then hyperthermia or hyponatremia is likely. LH, lightheadedness.

Table 1
Work-up of syncope and collapse

	Neurally Mediated or Nonarrhythmic	Postexertion Collapse	Hyperthermia and Hyponatremia	Arrhythmic	Seizure
Situational factors	Fear, fright, dehydration, upright posture	After extreme exertion	Hot weather, extreme exertion, excessive water intake	Exertional, unrelated to posture	Occasional, triggered by flickering or flashing lights
Prodrome	Lightheadedness, warmth, nausea	Fatigue, dizziness	Confusion, delirium	None or brief lightheadedness	Visual and auditory auras
Event characteristics	Slump to the ground, injury unusual	Slump to the ground, injury unusual	Subacute onset, could be simple fainting vs tonic-clonic seizure	Acute loss of consciousness, injury common, brief (<15 s), myoclonic jerks after collapse	Motor activity simultaneous with syncope, injury common, may last several minutes to hours
Postsyncope symptoms	Fatigue, nausea	Fatigue	Confusion, delirium	Usually none	Postictal state, confusion, urinary or stool incontinence, tongue biting, Todd paralysis
Number of episodes	Multiple	Few	Few	Few or 1	Many
Underlying disease	Unusual	Unusual	Unusual	Heart disease common	Neurologic disease common

occurs within 5 to 10 seconds of blood flow interruption to the brain; this is often described as a cardiac seizure. Seizure disorders have simultaneous loss of consciousness and motor disorder; however, this subtlety is often difficult to ascertain in clinical practice. Most of the syncope disorders have a short duration of unconsciousness; the exceptions are psychogenic syncope and seizures.

After syncope

Patients with NMS usually have continued symptoms of nausea, warmth, and fatigue after they awake. The fatigue can be last long enough that they do not feel well until they have slept. Patients with postexertion collapse and hyperthermia/hyponatremia also have continued symptoms such as fatigue and delirium, which tend to be even more profound than in those with NMS. In contrast, patients with cardiac syncope generally feel well immediately on regaining consciousness, so much so that they often refuse medical attention. After seizures, patients usually gradually awaken and clear their sensorium. Confusion about how the athlete came to be on the ground is normal; postictal confusion is a more profound and global confusion, so much so that they are not even aware that they are on the ground. Vital signs, including orthostatic vital signs, are a critical component of the work-up; NMS, seizures, and most cardiac syncope have normal vital signs. However, the presence of hypotension or bradycardia may denote dehydration or cardiac bradycardia.

Further Work-up and Management

Most patients with classic NMS require no further work-up, whereas the other forms of syncope are generally more concerning and require additional testing. Management is based on the underlying cardiac disease, and syncope is a marker for SCD in many of the cardiomyopathies (**Table 2**).

Electrocardiography

An ECG is critical for the diagnosis of bradyarrhythmias, although bradyarrhythmias can be transient and thus not seen on the initial ECG. ECG changes can suggest or diagnose the Brugada syndrome and LQTS. Placement of the right precordial leads in the second intercostal space can increase the sensitivity of the ECG for detecting a Brugada phenotype in some patients. In patients with suspected Brugada, long QT, or CPVT whose resting ECGs are normal, a drug challenge may unmask the ECG abnormalities. Sodium channel blockers such as flecainide and procainamide increase the ECG abnormalities of Brugada syndrome.[38,41] In long QT, beta agonists such as epinephrine and isoproterenol can also be useful in making the diagnosis. These agents would normally shorten the QT interval in normal individuals; however, in patients with long QT, prolongation of the corrected QT occurs.[44–46] Isoproterenol infusion can also be effective in triggering CPVT.

ECGs are abnormal in 90% of patients with hypertrophic cardiomyopathy.[22] ECG findings include ST segment depression, deep T-wave inversion, left axis deviation, and abnormal Q waves. In ARVC, ECG abnormalities include T-wave inversions in leads V1 to V3, epsilon waves and prolonged QRS in V1, and prolonged QRS complex in V1 of greater than 110 miliseconds.[25] Signal averaged electrocardiogram (SAECG) is abnormal in most patients with ARVC.[25]

Echocardiography

Increased LV wall thickness (>13–15 mm with no other cause for LVH), systolic anterior motion of the mitral valve, and LV outflow tract gradients can all be seen in HCM.[22] Echo findings in ARVC include an enlarged hypokinetic right ventricle with a thin right ventricular (RV) free wall and heavy RV trabeculations with a hyperreflective moderator band and occasional sacculations.[25] Echocardiography is typically normal in CPVT, LQTS, commotio cordis, and anomalous coronary arteries.

Magnetic Resonance Imaging

Magnetic resonance imaging (MRI) is sensitive in detecting increases in LV wall thickness in patients with HCM. MRI is particularly useful in detecting apical HCM. MRI was better than echocardiography in its ability to detect HCM in the anterolateral LV free wall as well as estimating the degree of hypertrophy in the basal anterolateral free wall. Late myocardial enhancement following gadolinium injection can aid in the diagnosis of HCM and may be a risk factor for SCD.[47] In ARVC, MRI can also show fatty infiltration and thinning of the RV free wall. It can also identify regional or global dilatation of the right ventricle and evaluate for late gadolinium enhancement but it is no longer the gold standard for ARVC.[25,48] Although patients with RVOT VT are said to have structurally normal hearts, particularly by echo, some studies suggest that there may be focal thinning and fatty replacement of the RVOT.

Exercise Treadmill Testing

Exercise treadmill testing (ETT) is valuable in reproducing a patient's symptoms and detecting

Table 2
Management of cardiac causes of syncope

Condition	Management	Sport Participation
Bradyarrhythmias (symptomatic sinus bradycardia, heart block)	Permanent pacemaker	No specific recommendations
HCM	LVOT obstruction[22]: • β-Blockers • Nondihydropyridine calcium channel blocker • Disopyramide Septal myectomy or alcohol septal ablation in symptomatic patients refractory to medical therapy Arrhythmia: ICD indications[22,56,57] • Secondary prevention of SCD • Family history of SCD • Syncope, not attributed to another cause • NSVT • Abnormal blood pressure response to exercise • Massive LVH (≥30 mm)	BC#36[56] Phenotypically (+): Exclusion from sport Genotypically (+), phenotypically (−): Can participate in sport ESC[58]: Phenotypically (+): Exclusion from sport Genotypically (+), phenotypically (−): Exclusion from all competitive sport
ARVC	ICD indications[53,59,60]. • Secondary prevention of SCD in patients who have had sustained VT or VF • Those with extensive disease • Syncope	Exclusion from sport
Coronary anomalies	Reimplantation of the anomalous coronary in the correct sinus or unroofing the myocardium that covers the intramyocardial segment	Exclusion from sports, but may resume if a normal stress study is obtained 3 mo after successful corrective surgery
Commotio cordis	ACLS management of acute ventricular arrhythmia	—

Condition	Treatment	Recommendations
Long QT syndrome	LQT1: β-blockers LQT2: β-blockers may be beneficial LQT3: possibly mexilitine	BC#36: Men with QT >470 ms and woman with >480 ms should be excluded from competitive sport Genotype (+), phenotype (−) can participate in sport ESC: Men with QT >440 ms and women with >460 ms and genotype (+) should be excluded from competitive sport Genotype (+), phenotype (−) are discouraged from participating in competitive sport
Brugada syndrome	Symptomatic patients with type 1 Brugada ECG (either spontaneously or after sodium channel blockade) who present with aborted SCD should receive an ICD Similar patients presenting with related symptoms such as syncope, seizure, or nocturnal agonal respiration should also undergo ICD implantation Asymptomatic patients[38,54]: the role of EPS is controversial	BC#36: Phenotype (+) patients (even only with symptoms) should be excluded from sport Patients who are genotype (+) phenotype (−), including a negative EP study, can participate in sport ESC: All patients should be excluded from competitive sport
RVOT VT	Adenosine (6–24 mg IV) is effective in acute termination β-Blockers Verapamil Radiofrequency ablation for definitive management (90% cure rates)	—
CPVT	β-Blockers ICD in most patients[41,61]	BC#36: Phenotype (+) patients (even only with symptoms) should be excluded from sport Genotype (+) phenotype (−) patients (including a negative EPS) can participate in sport ESC: All patients should be excluded from competitive sport

BC#36 and ESC agree that all patients with ICD should be excluded from competitive sport.

Abbreviations: ACLS, advanced cardiac life support; ARVC, arrhythmogenic right ventricular cardiomyopathy; BC#36, Bethesda Conference #36 recommendations; ESC, European Society of Cardiology recommendations; ICD, implantable cardioverter-defibrillator; IV, intravenous; LQT, long QT; LVOT, LV outflow tract; NSVT, nonsustained VT; VF, ventricular fibrillation.

ventricular arrhythmias during exertion. CPVT may be induced during ETT, and the severity of the tachycardia is directly related to the degree of exertion. RVOT VT can also be reproduced during ETT. Exercise testing may show induced ischemia in those with anomalous coronary arteries. During exercise, young adults and children should shorten their QT intervals. In patients with long QT, exercise stress testing may be useful because their QTs often fail to shorten or even prolong. Patients with LQT1 have diminished shortening of the QT interval and a reduced chronotropic response during exercise, followed by exaggerated lengthening of the QT interval as the heart rate declines during recovery after exercise. Patients with LQT2 have marked QT interval shortening and a normal chronotropic response during exercise. There is exaggerated lengthening of the QT interval as the heart rate declines during late recovery, described as after 4 minutes of exercise. Patients with LQT3 have a more marked decrease in the QT interval with exercise than either patients with LQT2 or controls.[49,50]

Cardiac Catheterization/Computed Tomography Angiograph

RV angiography can aid in the diagnosis of ARVC. The right ventricle is seen as dilated, often with trabeculae, some of which are transversely arranged and hypertrophic, and some of which are coarse in the apical region distal to the moderator band. Cardiac catheterization is also useful in the diagnosis of anomalous coronary arteries, although computed tomography (CT) angiography has generally supplanted cardiac catheterization.[51]

Electrophysiology Study

Electrophysiologic testing is rarely useful or needed, with the possible exception of ARVC and Brugada syndrome, although its use in both of these diagnoses is controversial.[52] In ARVC, early studies showed that electrophysiology study (EPS) may be useful in predicting future ventricular arrhythmias, but later studies have generally not replicated the early studies.[53] In Brugada syndrome, earlier studies have shown predictive value, whereas a later prospective study did not.[54]

Genetic Testing

Targeted genetic testing for the diagnosis of an individual may occasionally be useful, but, in general, should rarely be performed. In gray areas of diagnosis, genetic testing is predominantly useful in the LQTS, in which 75% to 80% are positive, and possibly the Brugada syndrome, in which 15% to 20% of individuals are positive. The primary use of genetic testing is in the management of family members.[55]

SUMMARY

Syncope in the athlete is especially concerning if it occurs during exertion, occurs without preceding symptoms, or if injury occurs. The work-up for syncope should focus on the history and vital signs, because these guide the diagnosis and indicate whether further testing is necessary. Ancillary tests such as ECGs, echocardiograms, and specific testing should be targeted based on the history.

REFERENCES

1. Link MS, Estes NA 3rd. How to manage athletes with syncope. Cardiol Clin 2007;25:457–66, vii.
2. Moya A, Sutton R, Ammirati F, et al. Guidelines for the diagnosis and management of syncope (version 2009). Eur Heart J 2009;30:2631–71.
3. Benditt DG, Nguyen JT. Syncope: therapeutic approaches. J Am Coll Cardiol 2009;53:1741–51.
4. Grubb BP. Clinical practice. Neurocardiogenic syncope. N Engl J Med 2005;352:1004–10.
5. Grubb BP, Temesy-Armos PN, Samoil D, et al. Tilt table testing in the evaluation and management of athletes with recurrent exercise-induced syncope. Med Sci Sports Exerc 1993;25:24–8.
6. Sneddon JF, Scalia G, Ward DE, et al. Exercise induced vasodepressor syncope. Br Heart J 1994; 71:554–7.
7. Calkins H, Seifert M, Morady F. Clinical presentation and long-term follow-up of athletes with exercise-induced vasodepressor syncope. Am Heart J 1995;129:1159–64.
8. Sakaguchi S, Shultz JJ, Remole SC, et al. Syncope associated with exercise, a manifestation of neurally mediated syncope. Am J Cardiol 1995; 75:476–81.
9. Kosinski D, Grubb BP, Kip K, et al. Exercise-induced neurocardiogenic syncope. Am Heart J 1996;132: 451–2.
10. Levine BD, Lane LD, Buckey JC, et al. Left ventricular pressure-volume and Frank-Starling relations in endurance athletes. Implications for orthostatic tolerance and exercise performance. Circulation 1991;84:1016–23.
11. Childress MA, O'Connor FG, Levine BD. Exertional collapse in the runner: evaluation and management in fieldside and office-based settings. Clin Sports Med 2010;29:459–76.
12. Roberts WO. A 12-yr profile of medical injury and illness for the Twin Cities Marathon. Med Sci Sports Exerc 2000;32:1549–55.

13. Holtzhausen LM, Noakes TD, Kroning B, et al. Clinical and biochemical characteristics of collapsed ultra-marathon runners. Med Sci Sports Exerc 1994;26:1095–101.

14. Rosner MH, Kirven J. Exercise-associated hyponatremia. Clin J Am Soc Nephrol 2007;2:151–61.

15. Armstrong LE, Epstein Y, Greenleaf JE, et al. American College of Sports Medicine position stand. Heat and cold illnesses during distance running. Med Sci Sports Exerc 1996;28:i–x.

16. Marsh SA, Jenkins DG. Physiological responses to the menstrual cycle: implications for the development of heat illness in female athletes. Sports Med 2002;32:601–14.

17. Noakes TD. A modern classification of the exercise-related heat illnesses. J Sci Med Sport 2008;11:33–9.

18. Speedy DB, Rogers IR, Noakes TD, et al. Exercise-induced hyponatremia in ultradistance triathletes is caused by inappropriate fluid retention. Clin J Sport Med 2000;10:272–8.

19. Colivicchi F, Ammirati F, Santini M. Epidemiology and prognostic implications of syncope in young competing athletes. Eur Heart J 2004;25:1749–53.

20. Stein R, Medeiros CM, Rosito GA, et al. Intrinsic sinus and atrioventricular node electrophysiologic adaptations in endurance athletes. J Am Coll Cardiol 2002;39:1033–8.

21. Maron BJ. Distinguishing hypertrophic cardiomyopathy from athlete's heart physiological remodelling: clinical significance, diagnostic strategies and implications for preparticipation screening. Br J Sports Med 2009;43:649–56.

22. Gersh BJ, Maron BJ, Bonow RO, et al. 2011 ACCF/AHA guideline for the diagnosis and treatment of hypertrophic cardiomyopathy: executive summary: a report of the American College of Cardiology Foundation/American Heart Association Task Force on Practice Guidelines. Circulation 2011;124:2761–96.

23. Basso C, Corrado D, Marcus FI, et al. Arrhythmogenic right ventricular cardiomyopathy. Lancet 2009;373:1289–300.

24. Dalal D, Nasir K, Bomma C, et al. Arrhythmogenic right ventricular dysplasia: a United States experience. Circulation 2005;112:3823–32.

25. Marcus FI, McKenna WJ, Sherrill D, et al. Diagnosis of arrhythmogenic right ventricular cardiomyopathy/dysplasia: proposed modification of the task force criteria. Circulation 2010;121:1533–41.

26. Maron BJ. Sudden death in young athletes. N Engl J Med 2003;349:1064–75.

27. Berbarie RF, Dockery WD, Johnson KB, et al. Use of multislice computed tomographic coronary angiography for the diagnosis of anomalous coronary arteries. Am J Cardiol 2006;98:402–6.

28. Basso C, Maron BJ, Corrado D, et al. Clinical profile of congenital coronary artery anomalies with origin from the wrong aortic sinus leading to sudden death in young competitive athletes. J Am Coll Cardiol 2000;35:1493–501.

29. Maron BJ, Estes NA 3rd. Commotio cordis. N Engl J Med 2010;362:917–27.

30. Solberg E, Embra B, Borjesson M, et al. Commotio cordis – under-recognized in Europe? A case report and review. Eur J Cardiovasc Prev Rehabil 2011;18:378–83.

31. Link MS. Commotio cordis: ventricular fibrillation triggered by chest impact-induced abnormalities in repolarization. Circ Arrhythm Electrophysiol 2012;5:425–32.

32. Madias C, Maron BJ, Alsheikh-Ali AA, et al. Commotio cordis. Indian Pacing Electrophysiol J 2007;7:235–45.

33. Link MS, Wang PJ, Pandian NG, et al. An experimental model of sudden death due to low-energy chest-wall impact (commotio cordis). N Engl J Med 1998;338:1805–11.

34. Alsheikh-Ali AA, Madias C, Supran S, et al. Marked variability in susceptibility to ventricular fibrillation in an experimental commotio cordis model. Circulation 2010;122:2499–504.

35. Goldenberg I, Moss AJ. Long QT syndrome. J Am Coll Cardiol 2008;51:2291–300.

36. Kapetanopoulos A, Kluger J, Maron BJ, et al. The congenital long QT syndrome and implications for young athletes. Med Sci Sports Exerc 2006;38:816–25.

37. Maron BJ, Doerer JJ, Haas TS, et al. Sudden deaths in young competitive athletes: analysis of 1866 deaths in the United States, 1980-2006. Circulation 2009;119:1085–92.

38. Antzelevitch C, Brugada P, Borggrefe M, et al. Brugada syndrome: report of the second consensus conference: endorsed by the Heart Rhythm Society and the European Heart Rhythm Association. Circulation 2005;111:659–70.

39. Lerman BB, Belardinelli L, West GA, et al. Adenosine-sensitive ventricular tachycardia: evidence suggesting cyclic AMP-mediated triggered activity. Circulation 1986;74:270–80.

40. Buxton AE, Marchlinski FE, Doherty JU, et al. Repetitive, monomorphic ventricular tachycardia: clinical and electrophysiologic characteristics in patients with and patients without organic heart disease. Am J Cardiol 1984;54:997–1002.

41. Napolitano C, Bloise R, Monteforte N, et al. Sudden cardiac death and genetic ion channelopathies: long QT, Brugada, short QT, catecholaminergic polymorphic ventricular tachycardia, and idiopathic ventricular fibrillation. Circulation 2012;125:2027–34.

42. Cerrone M, Napolitano C, Priori SG. Catecholaminergic polymorphic ventricular tachycardia: a paradigm to understand mechanisms of arrhythmias

associated to impaired Ca(2+) regulation. Heart Rhythm 2009;6:1652–9.

43. Leenhardt A, Lucet V, Denjoy I, et al. Catecholaminergic polymorphic ventricular tachycardia in children. A 7-year follow-up of 21 patients. Circulation 1995;91:1512–9.

44. Clur SA, Chockalingam P, Filippini LH, et al. The role of the epinephrine test in the diagnosis and management of children suspected of having congenital long QT syndrome. Pediatr Cardiol 2010;31:462–8.

45. Vyas H, Hejlik J, Ackerman MJ. Epinephrine QT stress testing in the evaluation of congenital long-QT syndrome: diagnostic accuracy of the paradoxical QT response. Circulation 2006;113:1385–92.

46. Krahn AD, Healey JS, Chauhan V, et al. Systematic assessment of patients with unexplained cardiac arrest: Cardiac Arrest Survivors With Preserved Ejection Fraction Registry (CASPER). Circulation 2009;120:278–85.

47. Harrigan CJ, Peters DC, Gibson CM, et al. Hypertrophic cardiomyopathy: quantification of late gadolinium enhancement with contrast-enhanced cardiovascular MR imaging. Radiology 2011;258: 128–33.

48. Sen-Chowdhry S, Prasad SK, Syrris P, et al. Cardiovascular magnetic resonance in arrhythmogenic right ventricular cardiomyopathy revisited: comparison with task force criteria and genotype. J Am Coll Cardiol 2006;48:2132–40.

49. Obeyesekere MN, Klein GJ, Modi S, et al. How to perform and interpret provocative testing for the diagnosis of Brugada syndrome, long-QT syndrome, and catecholaminergic polymorphic ventricular tachycardia. Circ Arrhythm Electrophysiol 2011;4: 958–64.

50. Horner JM, Horner MM, Ackerman MJ. The diagnostic utility of recovery phase QTc during treadmill exercise stress testing in the evaluation of long QT syndrome. Heart Rhythm 2011;8:1698–704.

51. Shriki JE, Shinbane JS, Rashid MA, et al. Identifying, characterizing, and classifying congenital anomalies of the coronary arteries. Radiographics 2012;32: 453–68.

52. Link MS, Estes NA. Athletes and arrhythmias. J Cardiovasc Electrophysiol 2010;21:1184–9.

53. Corrado D, Calkins H, Link MS, et al. Prophylactic implantable defibrillator in patients with arrhythmogenic right ventricular cardiomyopathy/dysplasia and no prior ventricular fibrillation or sustained ventricular tachycardia. Circulation 2010; 122:1144–52.

54. Priori SG, Gasparini M, Napolitano C, et al. Risk stratification in Brugada syndrome: results of the PRELUDE (PRogrammed ELectrical stimUlation preDictive valuE) registry. J Am Coll Cardiol 2012; 59:37–45.

55. Ackerman MJ, Priori SG, Willems S, et al. HRS/EHRA expert consensus statement on the state of genetic testing for the channelopathies and cardiomyopathies: this document was developed as a partnership between the Heart Rhythm Society (HRS) and the European Heart Rhythm Association (EHRA). Heart Rhythm 2011;8:1308–39.

56. Maron BJ, Ackerman MJ, Nishimura RA, et al. Task Force 4: HCM and other cardiomyopathies, mitral valve prolapse, myocarditis, and Marfan syndrome. J Am Coll Cardiol 2005;45:1340–5.

57. Maron BJ, Spirito P, Shen WK, et al. Implantable cardioverter-defibrillators and prevention of sudden cardiac death in hypertrophic cardiomyopathy. JAMA 2007;298:405–12.

58. Pelliccia A, Fagard R, Bjornstad HH, et al. Recommendations for competitive sports participation in athletes with cardiovascular disease: a consensus document from the Study Group of Sports Cardiology of the Working Group of Cardiac Rehabilitation and Exercise Physiology and the Working Group of Myocardial and Pericardial Diseases of the European Society of Cardiology. Eur Heart J 2005;26: 1422–45.

59. Boldt LH, Haverkamp W. Arrhythmogenic right ventricular cardiomyopathy: diagnosis and risk stratification. Herz 2009;34:290–7.

60. Corrado D, Leoni L, Link MS, et al. Implantable cardioverter-defibrillator therapy for prevention of sudden death in patients with arrhythmogenic right ventricular cardiomyopathy/dysplasia. Circulation 2003;108:3084–91.

61. Napolitano C, Priori SG. Diagnosis and treatment of catecholaminergic polymorphic ventricular tachycardia. Heart Rhythm 2007;4:675–8.

Exercise-Induced Arrhythmogenic Right Ventricular Cardiomyopathy
Seek and You Will Find

Andre La Gerche, MBBS, PhD[a,b],
Hein Heidbuchel, MD, PhD[a,*]

KEYWORDS

- Athlete • Right ventricle • Arrhythmias • Athlete's heart
- Arrhythmogenic right ventricular cardiomyopathy • Myocardial fibrosis • Endurance • Exercise

KEY POINTS

- Exercise-induced right ventricular cardiomyopathy refers to the observation that, among endurance athletes, ventricular arrhythmias are frequently associated with electrical, structural, and functional changes of the right ventricle (RV).
- Strenuous exercise exerts an increased hemodynamic load (wall stress, work, and oxygen demand), which is proportionally greater for the RV than for the left ventricle (LV). When this exercise load is sustained, evidence of myocardial injury also disproportionately affects the RV.
- Data from animal models (and some data in humans) raise the possibility that habitual intense exercise may lead to chronic fibrotic and proarrhythmic remodeling of the RV, and not the LV.
- Some athletes presenting with RV arrhythmias are at risk of sudden cardiac death even when presenting with seemingly mild symptoms.
- Proarrhythmic RV remodeling in athletes does not seem to be explained by the same genetic factors as familial arrhythmogenic RV cardiomyopathy. However, it may be caused by a combination of extreme exercise and a milder genetic predisposition, which is yet to be determined, or can be explained by extreme exercise associated with differential pulmonary circulatory conditions in different individuals.
- Greater awareness of this speculative entity may lead to greater recognition, pathophysiologic insights, and, ultimately, better treatment strategies.

INTRODUCTION

Exercise-induced arrhythmogenic right ventricular cardiomyopathy (EIARVC) refers to the observation that, among endurance athletes, ventricular arrhythmias most frequently arise from the right ventricle (RV) and are frequently associated with structural and functional changes of the RV. The arising phenotype is similar, if not indistinguishable, from the clinical spectrum of familial arrhythmogenic right ventricular cardiomyopathy (ARVC). Understanding of the interplay between genetic and environmental factors in the causation of ARVC is incomplete, and evolving evidence shows that strenuous exercise may accelerate disease

Funding and Potential Conflicts of Interest: See last page of article.
a Department of Cardiovascular Medicine, University Hospital Leuven, Herestraat 49, Leuven B-3000, Belgium;
b Department of Medicine, St Vincent's Hospital, University of Melbourne, 29 Regent Street, Fitzroy, Melbourne, VIC 3065, Australia
* Corresponding author. Director of Electrophysiology, University Hospital Gasthuisberg, Herestraat 49, Leuven B-3000, Belgium.
E-mail address: Hein.Heidbuchel@uz.kuleuven.ac.be

Card Electrophysiol Clin 5 (2013) 97–105
http://dx.doi.org/10.1016/j.ccep.2012.11.001
1877-9182/13/$ – see front matter © 2013 Elsevier Inc. All rights reserved.

progression in patients with an underlying genetic predisposition. The authors' observations extend this premise one stage further. They suggest that in endurance athletes undertaking extreme amounts of exercise over many years, the repeated transient excess in wall stress leads to structural and functional remodeling of the RV, which may create a substrate for arrhythmias in the absence of a known genetic predisposition. However, known mutations in desmosomal proteins account for approximately 50% of familial ARVC, and therefore it is plausible that a condition is being observed that is underpinned by a genetic predisposition (a mutation or combination of polymorphisms) that is yet to be discovered. Nevertheless, in contrast to familial forms of ARVC, the phenotype does not develop in the absence of intense sports conditioning. Another possibility is that the predisposition for EIARVC is not defined by the genetic makeup of the heart but by the specifics of the cardiopulmonary circulation. What is most immediately clinically relevant is that the RV should be considered a point of greatest stress in the heart of endurance athletes and should be the focus of investigations in athletes presenting with palpitations, arrhythmias, or syncope. The authors suspect that with awareness, this condition will be increasingly recognized, thus enabling refinement of treatment and prevention strategies.

WHAT IS EIARVC?

Heidbuchel and colleagues[1] coined the term *EIARVC* after observing that among endurance athletes, ventricular arrhythmias were frequently associated with electrical, structural and functional changes of the RV, and rarely of the left ventricle (LV). A comprehensive evaluation was undertaken on 46 high-level endurance athletes (performing $\geq 3 \times 2$ hours of sports per week for more than 5 years; 80% competitive; 80% cyclists) who had been diagnosed with sustained or nonsustained ventricular tachycardia or frequent ventricular ectopy (37%, 52%, and 11% of cases, respectively) in the context of nonspecific symptoms, such as palpitations and dizziness. Most ventricular arrhythmias (VAs) were of RV origin (86% of cases), which was surprising given that inherited cardiomyopathies, ischemic heart disease (from congenital coronary anomalies or atherosclerosis), and myocarditis are most frequently associated with VA and sudden cardiac death in young athletic cohorts.[2–4] Most of these pathologies would imply a left ventricular or biventricular substrate, contrasting with the high prevalence of RV pathology, which could only be explained by a major selection

bias resulting in athletes with familial ARVC being disproportionately represented. However, this bias did not seem likely and was not supported by the fact that only 1 athlete (2%) had a family history suggestive of ARVC. Rather, Heidbuchel and colleagues[1] proposed that the association between RV abnormalities and endurance sport practice could be better explained if it were endurance sport itself that was contributing to the creation of an arrhythmic substrate in the RV. In other words, the unifying feature of the cohort (the very high volume of sport practice) was the likely explanation for the unexpectedly high prevalence of RV abnormalities.

The second crucial finding from this study was that although the athletes frequently presented with nonspecific and mild symptoms, the arrhythmic outcome had an ominous course. After a medium follow-up of 4.7 years, 18 of 46 athletes had a major rhythm disorder, among whom 9 experienced (aborted) sudden death (all cyclists; a mean of 3 years after presentation).[1] Only an electrophysiologic study inducing reentrant arrhythmias was predictive for later arrhythmic events outcome (relative risk, 3.4; $P = .02$), indicating an underlying structural substrate. Among persons with VA, the prognosis in those without structural heart disease is generally excellent,[5,6] and this premise is thought to include the structural changes related to sports training ("athlete's heart"), which are considered a nonarrhythmogenic physiologic form of remodeling.[7] However, the distinction between athlete's heart and subtle RV dysfunction may be critical. Heidbuchel and colleagues[1] showed that even mild RV dysfunction could be the harbinger of a serious proarrhythmic substrate, thus emphasizing the need for a comprehensive assessment of the "forgotten" RV in endurance athletes.

To further validate the hypothesis that RV dysfunction was associated with a proarrhythmic state in the endurance athlete's heart, Ector and colleagues[8] performed a detailed quantitative RV angiographic evaluation in 22 high-level endurance athletes presenting with VAs, and compared the results with age- and sex-matched comparable athletes (n = 15) and nonathletes (n = 10). Although 27% of the athletes with arrhythmias had definite task force criteria for ARVC, evidence of an underlying familial predisposition was again uncommon (9%). Four different software algorithms were used to measure RV and LV volumes and ejection fraction from biplane RV angiography. All athletes had normal LV function. Athletes with arrhythmias had a small but highly significantly lower RV ejection fraction than athletes without arrhythmias and controls (49.1% vs 63.7% vs 67%, respectively; $P<.001$).[8] This decrease is clearly less pronounced than what is known from familial series of ARVC, but again indicates underlying structural changes in the RV that may be associated with the observed arrhythmogenicity. Many of these ventriculograms, when evaluated qualitatively by an experienced evaluator, were labeled as "normal for athlete's heart," indicating the importance of quantitative evaluation as stated in the revised ARVC task force criteria.[9] For the endurance athlete, the question remains as to why some athletes seemed to develop RV dysfunction.

THE RV IS THE ACHILLES HEEL OF THE ATHLETE'S HEART

The contribution of RV function to overall cardiac performance increases with exercise. At rest, the work requirement of the RV is minimal because of the very low RV afterload. However, with increasing exercise intensity, RV systolic pressures increase progressively,[10–18] and this translates into an increase in wall stress, coronary perfusion, and oxygen extraction, which is greater for the RV than the LV.[19,20]

Increases in RV Afterload and Work During Exercise

At rest, the RV pumps into a low-pressure, highly compliant pulmonary vasculature. Thus, little work is required of the RV at rest. RV mass and systolic pressure are approximately one-quarter to one-fifth those of the LV.[21] However, work requirements change significantly during exercise. Mean pulmonary arterial pressures (PAPs) are known to increase during exercise in healthy subjects,[14,15,22] and to an even greater extent in well-trained athletes.[16–18] A linear association between increases in cardiac output (CO) and PAP during exercise have been shown using invasive[11,14,22,23] and echocardiographic studies,[12,13] so that mean PAP will frequently exceed 30 mm Hg in athletes when CO exceeds 20 L/min. For example, Groves, Reeves and colleagues[17,18] reported invasively determined mean PAP values of up to 45 mm Hg ($\approx$ 75 mm Hg systolic PAP) in athletes, consistent with the authors' own echocardiographic estimates[12] and currently ongoing invasive study (La Gerche MD, PhD and Heidbuchel MD, PhD, 2012, unpublished data). An asymptote or plateau in PAP during higher-intensity exercise has not been observed. Rather, the greater the capacity for exercise, the greater the CO and the higher the PAP and RV load.

The Proportional Increase in RV Load Exceeds That of the LV During Exercise

Perhaps surprisingly, the relative contribution of the left and right ventricles to overall cardiac performance during exercise has seldom been investigated. However, current evidence in both animal and human studies is concordant in asserting that RV wall stress, work, and oxygen demand are less than for the LV at rest (as may be expected in the lower pressure system) but that the proportional increase in these measures during exercise is far greater for the RV. Hart and colleagues[24] instrumented the aorta and RV venous drainage of exercising dogs to determine RV oxygen extraction. At rest, oxygen extraction in the RV was approximately half that of the LV but then increased to a far greater extent during strenuous exercise so that oxygen extraction was similar in both ventricles.

This article's authors attempted to compare RV and LV hemodynamics during exercise using a combination of cardiac magnetic resonance (CMR) and echocardiographic measures to define end-systolic wall stress using the principles of the Laplace relationship.[20] Similar to the findings of Hart and colleagues[24] in exercising dogs, the authors found that RV load was approximately half that of the LV at rest, predominantly owing to the lower afterload pressures. However, during exercise, wall stress increased to a greater extent so that it approximated that of the LV during exercise (**Fig. 1**). This finding was caused by a greater proportional increase in systolic pressure, a greater increase in volume, and a lesser increase in systolic wall thickness. Furthermore, increases in RV wall stress were greater in endurance athletes than in nonathletes.

Prolonged Exercise-Induced RV Load Excess Leads to Disproportionate RV Dysfunction

It stands to reason that sustained excesses in RV wall stress, work, and oxygen demand may result in RV fatigue and/or damage. It has long been recognized that intense endurance exercise is associated with cardiac fatigue or injury, as evidenced by acute increases in troponin and B-type natriuretic peptide and decreases in cardiac function.[25] Multiple recent studies have assessed RV function after endurance exercise and have consistently reported decrements in RV function that are far more substantive than those observed for the LV.[26–29] Douglas and colleagues[30] showed that the RV dilated after an ultraendurance triathlon, whereas the LV dimensions were unchanged, and this observation was recently replicated using 2-dimensional and 3-dimensional echocardiographic measures.[26,28] It may be argued that echocardiographic assessment of RV function has significant limitations. However, studies using CMR imaging after intense endurance exercise

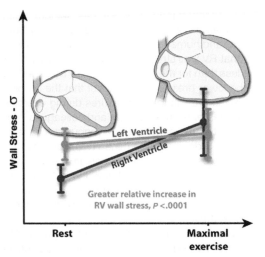

Fig. 1. Greater proportional increase in RV wall stress during exercise. Adapted from La Gerche and colleagues, who used a combination of echocardiographic and magnetic resonance imaging to show that, compared with the left ventricle, wall stress (a measure of afterload) was lower in the RV at rest but increased more during short intense exercise. (*Adapted from* La Gerche A, Heidbuchel H, Burns AT, et al. Disproportionate exercise load and remodeling of the athlete's right ventricle. Med Sci Sports Exerc 2011;43(6):974–81; with permission.)

have confirmed the same differential effects, with no change in LV function and a considerable reduction in RV ejection fraction.[31,32] Finally, although multiple studies have documented that no relationship exists between biomarkers of cardiac injury and changes in LV function,[25] La Gerche and colleagues[26] and other investigators[29] have documented moderately strong inverse correlations between the decrease in measures of RV function and the increase in release of troponin and B-type natriuretic peptide. Thus, it would seem reasonable to conclude that the RV is indeed the Achilles heel of the athlete's heart, whereby the RV bears the greatest increase in acute exercise load and the greatest injury after sustained exercise.

Chronic Remodeling of the Athlete's RV

Given the increasing RV demand during exercise, one could hypothesize that with increasing amounts of habitual exercise, the RV may remodel in an attempt to approximate the morphology and function of the LV. However, evidence of disproportionate RV remodeling in endurance athletes is conflicting. Scharhag and colleagues[33] described symmetric ventricular enlargement in 21 young endurance athletes (aged 27 ± 5 years), whereas in a slightly larger cohort, this article's authors found larger relative increases in the RV:LV ratio

for end-systolic volumes when comparing endurance athletes with healthy controls.[20] This finding could relate to the fact that the authors' cohort was older (aged 36 ± 8 years) and had greater exposure to exercise-induced load excess. However, firm conclusions are difficult to draw from these disparate results, especially considering that the degree of ventricular asymmetry resulting from exercise is likely to be slight. One could argue that all prior studies in athletic cohorts have been underpowered to assess subtle ventricular differences. This proposition is supported by the results of Aaron and colleagues,[34] who recruited a large cohort of 1867 nonathletes to show that the amount of strenuous activity predicted RV mass and volumes independent of LV size.

Furthermore, some parallel insights may be gained from animal experiments based on an induced aortocaval fistula in pigs.[35] This intervention leads to a chronic high-output cardiac state with an increase in volume and pressure load somewhat akin to exercise. After 3 months, a disproportionate increase occurred in RV stroke work index relative to that of the LV (+216% vs +70%), RV fibrosis, and the development of RV dysfunction. Compared with the more "physiologic" LV hypertrophy characterized by myocyte length increase and increased local production of insulin-like growth factor (IGF), the RV showed more pronounced hypertrophy, increase in both myocyte length and diameter, and associated increased collagen deposition. An increase also occurred in endothelin I and angiotensin II production. The authors postulated that the differential loads led to different gene expression and different structural changes.[35]

More recently, the Barcelona group of Lluis Mont and colleagues[36] established a rat model of endurance activity. Although rats can be forced to run only for a maximum of 1 hour per day (ie, much shorter than man), the running rats showed increased interstitial fibrosis in both atria and in the RV after 16 weeks, in contrast to none in the LV. This finding was associated with inducibility of ventricular arrhythmias in 42% of the exercise rats, versus only 6% in controls ($P = .05$). Cessation of exercise reversed the fibrotic changes. The question is whether fibrogenesis can also be prevented in man with much longer-standing exercise history. Moreover, it remains to be seen whether administration of an angiotensin-converting enzyme inhibitor or angiotensin receptor blocker could also lead to reversibility or prevention, offering further prospect for clinical medicine. However, no data are available so far on possible preventive or reversible effects of these drugs in athletes with supraventricular or ventricular arrhythmias.

Two recent studies have reported small patches of delayed gadolinium enhancement (DGE) on magnetic resonance studies in 13% and 50% of athletes with a longstanding history of endurance competition.[37,38] These findings could be consistent with the aforementioned animal models of sustained exercise excess resulting in chronic fibrous remodeling and arrhythmogenicity. However, several studies have failed to identify DGE in endurance athletes[31,32] and no studies have assessed the relationship between DGE and clinical events (such as arrhythmias) in athletes. Thus, it would be premature to suggest that patches of DGE represent a substrate for arrhythmias, although some investigators are drawing this link in cases of unexplained cardiac arrest in highly trained athletes.[39]

WHAT FACTORS PREDISPOSE AN ATHLETE TO DEVELOPING EXERCISE-INDUCED RV CARDIOMYOPATHY?

Although exercise may impose a greater demand on the RV, clearly not all athletes develop RV dysfunction at the end of an endurance event. Similarly, the RV structural remodeling of endurance athletes varies considerably despite similar training histories. Exercise-induced RV cardiomyopathy may represent the small fraction of athletes in whom RV remodeling is particularly profound or in whom the normal balance between cellular stress and repair is imperfect. No formal estimates exist regarding the proportion of athletes who develop RV tachyarrhythmias with or without RV dysfunction. Uncertainty exists regarding both the numerator (complete registry of cases?) and the denominator (population of intense endurance athletes at risk?). Rough estimates based on the referral pattern for the authors' tertiary care center and the number of registered competitive and high-level recreational cyclists in Belgium show that the yearly incidence for developing the phenotype may be approximately 1 in 1000 overall but may be 1 in 100 in international top-level athletes in the mentioned disciplines. Its relatively low prevalence is further highlighted by a normal survival curve in 119 former athletes participating in the Tour of Switzerland between 1975 and 1995; the observed survival was the same as that of a matched Swiss male population.[40] Nevertheless, the question remains as to which individual facilitating factors may play a role in developing exercise-induced ARVC.

Genetic Predisposition

As has been discussed at length, the authors contend that the hemodynamic stressors of exercise are a major factor influencing RV remodeling.

This environmental factor could be modulated by genetic factors, because desmosomal mutations and alterations are known to be the basis for familial ARVC. It is well established that exercise activity promotes the development of RV dysfunction and arrhythmogenicity in mutation carriers,[41,42] and a similar relationship was described recently for left cardiomyopathies caused by lamin A/C mutations.[43] Therefore, it is obvious to suspect that the similar phenotypes found in high-level athletes as in familial ARVC are caused by unmasking latent mutations. La Gerche and colleagues[44] systematically evaluated the 5 desmosomal genes for mutations (through sequencing) and larger genetic rearrangements (through multiplex ligation-dependent probe amplification) in a cohort of 47 athletes, of whom 87% had definite or probable criteria for an ARVC phenotype. The proportion with desmosomal mutations was much lower than that described for familial ARVC (13% vs ≈50%).[45–51] If RV arrhythmogenicity were the early expression of a latent underlying genetic (desmosomal) mutation, at least a similar prevalence as in familial forms would be expected. Moreover, familial ARVC was only present rarely (in 2/47 athletes).

Some have argued that a lower mutation rate might be seen in sporadic ARVC cases than in familial cohorts, and that this could explain the low mutation rate in the authors' cohort. However, most studies have recruited sporadic "index cases" through including unrelated cases as they present to the respective institutions. Because it is principally a familial disease, a proportion of index cases clearly have a positive family history (between 21% and 38%).[46,49–51] When analyzing the 4 largest studies that have included index cases with and without a positive family history, the mutation rate varies between 34% and 56% in index cases without a family history. In none of these studies does the rate of mutation differ between those with and without a family history.

Although other genetic predispositions cannot be excluded, the authors do not believe that exercise-induced ARVC is simply an unmasking of mutation-dependent familial ARVC. Their genetic findings strengthen their initial hypothesis that excessive strain on the RV by sports itself can be regarded as one side of a continuous spectrum in which myocardial integrity is perturbed because of a mismatch of strain and desmosomal integrity. With mutated desmosomes, normal levels of myocardial wall stress lead to cellular disruption and (fibrofatty) repair, ending in familial ARVC. But the authors propose that a similar phenotype may develop when excessive wall stress disrupts normal desmosomes, such as when the environmental factor plays the key role (**Fig. 2**). As in other diseases, polygenetic factors, many outside the desmosomes, may interplay with environmental factors (here: exercise) to result in a phenotype. The authors do not believe, however, that cardiac monogenetic traits are or need to be the sole explanation for individual susceptibility.

Illicit Drug Use

Performance-enhancing drugs are frequently cited as another potential confounder. Illicit drug use may be common in high-level endurance athletes, although no reliable data exist on its prevalence. However, for most modern performance-enhancing drugs, no direct cardiopathic effect has been described.[52] Moreover, if they were the direct cause, why they would selectively affect the RV is unclear. Amphetamines, for instance, are known to cause LV microinfarcts and scarring, with secondary arrhythmias that often originate in the LV. Therefore, the authors do not consider illicit drugs to be the direct cause. Their use may, however, be involved indirectly, such as through allowing longer and more strenuous endurance activity more frequently, thereby facilitating development of the phenotype.

PERSPECTIVES AND CLINICAL RELEVANCE

This article does not negate the clear fact that physical activity can reduce cardiovascular morbidity and mortality. Exercise is good and essential for all. However, one may have to realize that adaptation of the athlete's heart is not always able to accommodate the sustained hemodynamic loads placed on it (**Fig. 3**). In some, intense endurance activity can lead to cardiac sports injury in the form of supraventricular or ventricular arrhythmias. Although the number of data is increasing, the prevalence of life-threatening arrhythmic problems is definitely small. However, as with other sports injuries, recognizing the problem in an early phase can prevent disaster and may lead to measures that allow safe and enjoyable continuation of sports participation.

Diagnosis of RV arrhythmogenicity is not straightforward. Even in athletes with documented arrhythmias, confirming RV damage and proving compromised prognosis (ie, differentiating it from benign idiopathic RV outflow tract extrasystoles) is cumbersome. It requires an extensive workup with expert electrophysiologic insight. The diagnosis mainly resides on electrical findings (including an invasive electrophysiology study in some) rather

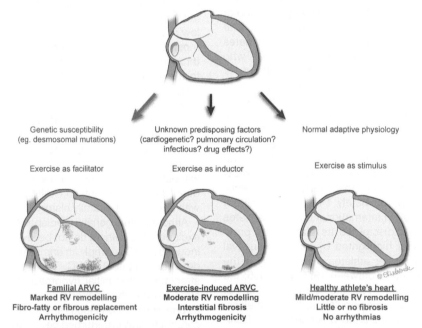

Fig. 2. Interaction between genetic and environmental factors may be required to create an ARVC-like phenotype. Familial ARVC is caused by an identifiable mutation in genes encoding various elements of cardiac structure (most commonly desmosomal proteins) combined with some environmental risk, such as exercise, which places physical stress on these weakened structures. The inverse may be true. Cardiac structure with a very mild alteration in structural integrity (largely unidentifiable with current genetic testing) may combine with marked physical stress from extreme exercise to cause a similar overall effect on myocardial structure. The "healthy athlete's heart" predicates that in the presence of favorable genetics, the heart may be able to better withstand the rigors of lifelong intense training.

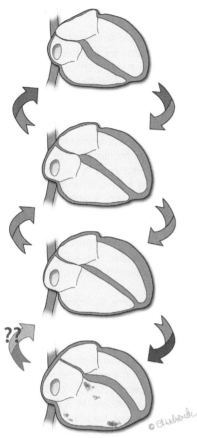

Normal training and recovery
Short-term hypertrophy and complete
regression following detraining

Sustained endurance training and recovery
Increasing cardiac remodelling (? particularly of the RV)
without complete regression following detraining

Chronic over-training with insufficient recovery
Pronounced remodelling (frequently RV > LV)
with limited regression following detraining

Increased risk of fibrosis, RV dysfunction and arrhythmias

Fig. 3. Healthy exercise training and recovery versus adverse cardiac remodeling after sustained overtraining. The orthodox view of the athlete's heart is that training results in symmetric hypertrophy of all cardiac chambers, which readily regresses with detraining ("normal training and recovery"). However, evolving evidence shows that sustained endurance training may lead to a degree of irreversible remodeling and, probably in a very small proportion of athletes, this may lead to more marked RV-dominant changes with an increased propensity to arrhythmias.

than imaging (with CMR normal in many athletes). However, physicians should be alert to suspicious symptoms (eg, exertional sudden dyspnea or light headedness) and findings, such as negative T waves beyond V_2, ventricular premature beats (VPB) with a left bundle branch morphology on electrocardiogram (especially when $\geq$2500 VPB are seen on a 24-hour Holter), or exercise-induced arrhythmias seen during an exercise test.

Much is yet to be determined. The data and hypotheses relating to exercise-induced RV cardiomyopathy are derived from only a few centers. The authors suspect that with greater awareness, the condition will be increasingly recognized. Validation in larger cohorts and from other centers will be important in validating this concept and will enable a better estimate of prevalence. Similarly, much remains to be learned about the way in which hemodynamic, genetic, and possibly other factors combine to explain why a minority of athletes are

affected. With better understanding will come the opportunity for better prevention and treatment strategies.

FUNDING AND POTENTIAL CONFLICTS OF INTEREST

Publication of this article was not funded.

Dr Heidbuchel is holder of the AstraZeneca Chair in Cardiac Electrophysiology, University of Leuven; received research funding through the University of Leuven from Siemens Medical Solutions; is Coordinating Clinical Investigator for the Biotronik-sponsored EuroEco study on health-economics of remote device monitoring; is a member of the scientific advisory board of Biosense Webster, Inc, St Jude Medical, Inc, Siemens Medical Solutions, Boehringer-Ingelheim, Bayer, and sanofi-aventis; and receives unconditional research grants through the University of Leuven from St Jude Medical, Medtronic, Biotronik, and Boston Scientific Inc.

Dr La Gerche receives a postdoctoral research scholarship from the Australian National Health and Medical Research Council.

REFERENCES

1. Heidbuchel H, Hoogsteen J, Fagard R, et al. High prevalence of right ventricular involvement in endurance athletes with ventricular arrhythmias. Role of an electrophysiologic study in risk stratification. Eur Heart J 2003;24(16):1473–80.

2. Corrado D, Basso C, Rizzoli G, et al. Does sports activity enhance the risk of sudden death in adolescents and young adults? J Am Coll Cardiol 2003; 42(11):1959–63.

3. Maron BJ, Doerer JJ, Haas TS, et al. Sudden deaths in young competitive athletes: analysis of 1866 deaths in the United States, 1980-2006. Circulation 2009;119(8):1085–92.

4. de Noronha SV, Sharma S, Papadakis M, et al. Aetiology of sudden cardiac death in athletes in the United Kingdom: a pathological study. Heart 2009; 95(17):1409–14.

5. Kennedy HL, Whitlock JA, Sprague MK, et al. Long-term follow-up of asymptomatic healthy subjects with frequent and complex ventricular ectopy. N Engl J Med 1985;312(4):193–7.

6. Bikkina M, Larson MG, Levy D. Prognostic implications of asymptomatic ventricular arrhythmias: the Framingham Heart Study. Ann Intern Med 1992; 117(12):990–6.

7. Prior DL, La Gerche A. The athlete's heart. Heart 2012;98(12):947–55.

8. Ector J, Ganame J, van der Merwe N, et al. Reduced right ventricular ejection fraction in endurance athletes presenting with ventricular arrhythmias: a quantitative angiographic assessment. Eur Heart J 2007;28(3):345–53.

9. Marcus FI, McKenna WJ, Sherrill D, et al. Diagnosis of arrhythmogenic right ventricular cardiomyopathy/dysplasia: proposed modification of the task force criteria. Eur Heart J 2010;31(7):806–14.

10. Stickland MK, Welsh RC, Haykowsky MJ, et al. Effect of acute increases in pulmonary vascular pressures on exercise pulmonary gas exchange. J Appl Phys 2006;100(6):1910–7.

11. Lewis GD, Murphy RM, Shah RV, et al. Pulmonary vascular response patterns during exercise in left ventricular systolic dysfunction predict exercise capacity and outcomes. Circ Heart Fail 2011;4(3): 276–85.

12. La Gerche A, MacIsaac AI, Burns AT, et al. Pulmonary transit of agitated contrast is associated with enhanced pulmonary vascular reserve and right ventricular function during exercise. J Appl Physiol 2010;109(5):1307–17.

13. Argiento P, Chesler N, Mule M, et al. Exercise stress echocardiography for the study of the pulmonary circulation. Eur Respir J 2010;35(6):1273–8.

14. Stanek V, Widimsky J, Degre S, et al. The lesser circulation during exercise in healthy subjects. Prog Respir Res 1975;9:295–315.

15. Naeije R, Chesler N. Pulmonary circulation at exercise. Comprehensive physiology, Vol. 2. New York: John Wiley & Sons, Inc; 2012. p. 711–41.

16. Bevegard S, Holmgren A, Jonsson B. Circulatory studies in well trained athletes at rest and during heavy exercise. With special reference to stroke volume and the influence of body position. Acta Physiol Scand 1963;57:26–50.

17. Groves BM, Reeves JT, Sutton JR, et al. Operation EVEREST II: elevated high-altitude pulmonary resistance unresponsive to oxygen. J Appl Physiol 1987; 63(2):521–30.

18. Reeves JT, Dempsey JA, Grover RF. Pulmonary circulation during exercise. In: Weir EK, Reeves JT, editors. Pulmonary vascular physiology and physiopathology. New York: Marcel Dekker; 1989. p. 107–33.

19. Zong P, Tune JD, Downey HF. Mechanisms of oxygen demand/supply balance in the right ventricle. Exp Biol Med (Maywood) 2005;230(8):507–19.

20. La Gerche A, Heidbuchel H, Burns AT, et al. Disproportionate exercise load and remodeling of the athlete's right ventricle. Med Sci Sports Exerc 2011; 43(6):974–81.

21. Jurcut R, Giusca S, La Gerche A, et al. The echocardiographic assessment of the right ventricle: what to do in 2010? Eur J Echocardiogr 2010;11(2):81–96.

22. Kovacs G, Berghold A, Scheidl S, et al. Pulmonary arterial pressure during rest and exercise in healthy subjects: a systematic review. Eur Respir J 2009; 34(4):888–94.

23. Stanek V, Jebavy P, Hurych J, et al. Central haemodynamics during supine exercise and pulmonary artery occlusion in normal subjects. Bull Physiopathol Respir (Nancy) 1973;9(5):1203–17.

24. Hart BJ, Bian X, Gwirtz PA, et al. Right ventricular oxygen supply/demand balance in exercising dogs. Am J Physiol Heart Circ Physiol 2001;281(2):H823–30.

25. Shave R, Baggish A, George K, et al. Exercise-induced cardiac troponin elevation: evidence, mechanisms, and implications. J Am Coll Cardiol 2010;56(3):169–76.

26. La Gerche A, Burns AT, Mooney DJ, et al. Exercise-induced right ventricular dysfunction and structural remodelling in endurance athletes. Eur Heart J 2012;33(8):998–1006.

27. La Gerche A, Connelly KA, Mooney DJ, et al. Biochemical and functional abnormalities of left and right ventricular function after ultra-endurance exercise. Heart 2008;94(7):860–6.

28. Oxborough D, Shave R, Warburton D, et al. Dilatation and dysfunction of the right ventricle immediately after ultraendurance exercise: exploratory insights from conventional two-dimensional and speckle tracking echocardiography. Circ Cardiovasc Imaging 2011; 4(3):253–63.

29. Neilan TG, Januzzi JL, Lee-Lewandrowski E, et al. Myocardial injury and ventricular dysfunction related to training levels among nonelite participants in the Boston marathon. Circulation 2006;114(22):2325–33.

30. Douglas PS, O'Toole ML, Hiller WD, et al. Different effects of prolonged exercise on the right and left ventricles. J Am Coll Cardiol 1990;15(1):64–9.

31. Mousavi N, Czarnecki A, Kumar K, et al. Relation of biomarkers and cardiac magnetic resonance imaging after marathon running. Am J Cardiol 2009;103(10): 1467–72.

32. Trivax JE, Franklin BA, Goldstein JA, et al. Acute cardiac effects of marathon running. J Appl Physiol 2010;108(5):1148–53.

33. Scharhag J, Schneider G, Urhausen A, et al. Athlete's heart: right and left ventricular mass and function in male endurance athletes and untrained individuals determined by magnetic resonance imaging. J Am Coll Cardiol 2002;40(10):1856–63.

34. Aaron CP, Tandri H, Barr RG, et al. Physical activity and right ventricular structure and function. The MESA-Right Ventricle Study. Am J Respir Crit Care Med 2011;183(3):396–404.

35. Modesti PA, Vanni S, Bertolozzi I, et al. Different growth factor activation in the right and left ventricles in experimental volume overload. Hypertension 2004;43(1):101–8.

36. Benito B, Gay-Jordi G, Serrano-Mollar A, et al. Cardiac arrhythmogenic remodeling in a rat model of long-term intensive exercise training. Circulation 2011;123(1):13–22.

37. Wilson M, O'Hanlon R, Prasad S, et al. Diverse patterns of myocardial fibrosis in lifelong, veteran endurance athletes. J Appl Physiol 2011;110(6): 1622–6.

38. La Gerche A, Burns AT, Mooney DJ, et al. Exercise-induced right ventricular dysfunction and structural remodelling in endurance athletes. Eur Heart J 2011;33(8):998–1006.

39. Trivax JE, McCullough PA. Phidippides cardiomyopathy: a review and case illustration. Clin Cardiol 2012;35(2):69–73.

40. Baldesberger S, Bauersfeld U, Candinas R, et al. Sinus node disease and arrhythmias in the long-term follow-up of former professional cyclists. Eur Heart J 2008;29(1):71–8.

41. Sen-Chowdhry S, Syrris P, Ward D, et al. Clinical and genetic characterization of families with arrhythmogenic right ventricular dysplasia/cardiomyopathy provides novel insights into patterns of disease expression. Circulation 2007;115(13):1710–20.

42. Kirchhof P, Fabritz L, Zwiener M, et al. Age- and training-dependent development of arrhythmogenic right ventricular cardiomyopathy in heterozygous plakoglobin-deficient mice. Circulation 2006;114(17): 1799–806.

43. Pasotti M, Klersy C, Pilotto A, et al. Long-term outcome and risk stratification in dilated cardiolaminopathies. J Am Coll Cardiol 2008;52(15):1250–60.

44. La Gerche A, Robberecht C, Kuiperi C, et al. Lower than expected desmosomal gene mutation prevalence in endurance athletes with complex ventricular arrhythmias of right ventricular origin. Heart 2010; 96(16):1268–74.

45. Sen-Chowdhry S, Syrris P, McKenna WJ. Role of genetic analysis in the management of patients with arrhythmogenic right ventricular dysplasia/cardiomyopathy. J Am Coll Cardiol 2007;50(19):1813–21.

46. Dalal D, Molin LH, Piccini J, et al. Clinical features of arrhythmogenic right ventricular dysplasia/cardiomyopathy associated with mutations in plakophilin-2. Circulation 2006;113(13):1641–9.

47. Gerull B, Heuser A, Wichter T, et al. Mutations in the desmosomal protein plakophilin-2 are common in arrhythmogenic right ventricular cardiomyopathy. Nat Genet 2004;36(11):1162–4.

48. Pilichou K, Nava A, Basso C, et al. Mutations in desmoglein-2 gene are associated with arrhythmogenic right ventricular cardiomyopathy. Circulation 2006;113(9):1171–9.

49. van Tintelen JP, Entius MM, Bhuiyan ZA, et al. Plakophilin-2 mutations are the major determinant of familial arrhythmogenic right ventricular dysplasia/cardiomyopathy. Circulation 2006;113(13):1650–8.

50. Fressart V, Duthoit G, Donal E, et al. Desmosomal gene analysis in arrhythmogenic right ventricular dysplasia/cardiomyopathy: spectrum of mutations and clinical impact in practice. Europace 2010; 12(6):861–8.

51. den Haan AD, Tan BY, Zikusoka MN, et al. Comprehensive desmosome mutation analysis in North Americans with arrhythmogenic right ventricular dysplasia/cardiomyopathy. Circ Cardiovasc Genet 2009;2(5):428–35.

52. Deligiannis A, Bjornstad H, Carre F, et al. ESC Study Group of Sports Cardiology Position Paper on adverse cardiovascular effects of doping in athletes. Eur J Cardiovasc Prev Rehabil 2006;13(5):687–94.

Bradyarrhythmias
How Slow Is Too Slow in the Athlete?

Ricardo Stein, ScD, MD*, Anderson Donelli da Silveira, MD

KEYWORDS

• Bradycardia • Athletic training • Sinus node • Aerobic exercise

KEY POINTS

- Sinus bradycardia is by far the most common bradyarrhythmia in the athlete.
- Sinus rates in the 30 to 40 beat per minute range are fairly common in the highly conditioned athlete.
- Endurance athletes present a higher prevalence of sinus bradycardia and AV conduction abnormalities, as a result of a high resting vagal tone, or significantly lower intrinsic heart rates.
- The training bradycardia seen in athletes is associated with an increased stroke volume. The cardiac output remains constant at rest and at submaximal workloads compared with sedentary controls.
- Unless associated with symptoms or with other arrthmyas, sinus bradycardia is a benign finding in the athlete.

INTRODUCTION

Athletic bradycardia is a nonpathologic condition commonly associated with aerobic exercise, especially identified in well-conditioned endurance athletes.[1] Since the beginning of the modern era Olympic Games, with the establishment of the marathon as an Olympic event, scientists and physicians have been studying the physiologic effects of endurance exercise in the cardiovascular system.[2] In the beginning of the twentieth century, the first observational studies had shown a slow pulse that has been confirmed by electrocardiography.[3–5]

It is well known that chronic exercise can lead to a series of morphologic and functional adaptations that are directly correlated to the type, duration, intensity, and years of practice.[6] Their clinical expression can be influenced by the genetic, humoral, and metabolic factors that vary individually. Since the second-half of the last century, alterations founded in athlete's electrocardiogram (ECG) have been considered an electrical expression of these adaptations.

Sinus bradycardia is by far the most common bradyarrhythmia in the athlete. It is correlated with the training level and can result in extremely low heart rates at rest.[7] Sinus pauses are also described, and can have more than 2 seconds of duration.[8] Sinus arrhythmia and wandering atrial pacemaker are also more prevalent in athletes compared with the general population.[9]

Atrioventricular (AV) delayed conduction is common and manifests electrocardiographically as first-degree AV blocks and type I second-degree AV blocks (Wenckebach phenomenon). Borderline PR intervals can be seen in up to one-third of trained endurance athletes.[9] Transient third-degree AV block and junctional escape beats can appear as a result of marked sinus bradycardia and delayed AV conduction. However, type II second- and third-degree AV blocks always should lead to a further investigation in chronic exercisers.

PATHOPHYSIOLOGY

In normal conditions there exists a well-balanced autonomic tone influencing the sinoatrial node,

Disclosures: No conflicts of interest to declare.
Cardiology Division, Hospital de Clínicas de Porto Alegre, Universidade Federal do Rio Grande do Sul, Rua Ramiro Barcelos 2350, Porto Alegre, Rio Grande do Sul 90035-007, Brazil
* Corresponding author. Cardiology Division, Hospital de Clínicas de Porto Alegre, Rua Ramiro Barcelos 2350, Porto Alegre, Rio Grande do Sul 90035–007, Brazil.
E-mail address: rstein@cardiol.br

with the sympathetic and parasympathetic systems having opposite effects on this natural pacemaker depolarization. A complex interrelation among different systems determines the autonomic tone at the sinoatrial node. There are cortical inputs to the medullary centers, and some visceral afferent inputs increase parasympathetic tone resulting in bradycardia.[10] Several reflexes are present for homeostasis. For example, the baroreflex is important in sensing changes in blood pressure, increasing or decreasing the heart rate by autonomic influences at the sinoatrial node to maintain appropriate cardiac output.[11]

Most peripheral factors that regulate heart rate can be uncovered by examining the physiologic changes delivered by training. Sigvardsson and colleagues[12] examined the role of the sympathetic nervous system in training-induced resting bradycardia with rats trained on treadmills comparing chemically sympathectomized animals with untreated control subjects. No training bradycardia was found in the sympathectomized group, although the untreated control subjects had a significant decrease in resting heart rate. The trained denervated hearts responded normally to adrenergic stimulation, implying that adrenergic sensitivity is not affected by the trained state.

The training bradycardia seen in athletes is associated with an increased stroke volume. Cardiac output remains constant at rest and at submaximal workloads compared with sedentary control subjects. Increased central vagal cholinergic drive and inhibitory mechanisms are believed to be involved in the bradycardia. However, whether the changes in the autonomic balance are intracardiac or peripheral was not clear. Clausen and coworkers[13,14] have done much to uncover the mechanism for training bradycardia by experiments involving various muscle groups, comparing trained and untrained limbs in the same subject. These studies have elicited that local skeletal muscle adaptation (increased muscle blood flow and induction of mitochondrial aerobic pathway enzymes) is restricted to the trained limb and, surprisingly, maximal oxygen consumption is increased while testing the trained limb but not the untrained limb. Relative bradycardia during exercise was observed only when exercising the trained limb, and the effect on heart rate was greater with leg muscle training than arm training.[14] The authors concluded that there were cardiac and peripheral effects from training acting through the autonomic nervous system.

Many studies have indicated that long-term endurance training increases parasympathetic activity and decreases sympathetic activity directed to the human heart at rest.[15–18] These exercise-induced autonomic alterations, allied with a possible reduction in intrinsic heart rate, decrease resting heart rate and increase heart rate variability at rest.[19–21] Some studies using autonomic blockade also found an increased parasympathetic control of heart rate after endurance training.[15,22] The training history of an athlete influences their physiologic response to exercise, and it is important to note that there are individual differences in response to exercise.[23]

The efferent sympathetic neural outflow to the sinoatrial node in the heart is reduced by exercise.[24] Smith and colleagues[25] showed that a change in baroreceptor sensitivity could be another possible mechanism contributing to exercise bradycardia. Detraining and bed rest studies also depicted the influence of training in autonomic function, as a study by Hughson and colleagues[26] reported a significant reduction in parasympathetic activity after 28 days of head-down bed rest.

In a meta-analysis, Sandercock and colleagues[27] studied the effect of exercise training in heart rate variability. They founded a significant effect of exercise training on resting RR interval and high-frequency power. This information supports current theory that aerobic exercise can alter neuroregulatory control over the heart and that changes in RR interval demonstrated that training induces a resting bradycardia accompanied by increased cardiac vagal modulation in healthy individuals. By this mechanism, one could also hypothesize that exercise training may be able to exert an antiarrhythmic effect.

Stein and colleagues[28] used transesophageal atrial stimulation to evaluate aerobically trained athletes and sedentary individuals to test the hypothesis that parasympathetic activity, as detected by heart rate variability, could be associated with changes in AV conduction. Athletes presented with Wenckebach AV node conduction at lower heart rates than those of sedentary individuals, suggesting a longer AV node refractory period. However, this could only be partially explained by increased parasympathetic activity (24%), as detected by a time domain index of heart rate variability, suggesting that nonautonomic factors could contribute to this change in AV conduction.

In the beginning of the new century, the same Brazilian study group performed an experiment with six aerobically trained athletes and six healthy individuals. All of them were male, had similar ages, and presented normal rest ECG.[29] The sinus cycle length, AV conduction intervals, sinus node recovery time, Wenckebach cycle, and anterograde effective refractory period of the AV node were evaluated by invasive electrophysiologic studies at baseline, after intravenous atropine, and after addition of intravenous propranolol. The sinus cycle length, Wenckebach cycle, and anterograde effective refractory period of the AV node were longer in athletes at baseline, after atropine, and after propranolol, demonstrating under double-pharmacologic blockade that sinus automaticity and AV node conduction changes of endurance athletes are related to intrinsic physiology and not to autonomic influences.

The physiologic mechanisms by which endurance training may induce these intrinsic changes in the specialized conduction system of the heart are unknown and may be multifactorial. An altered ionic balance across the membrane,[30] and biochemical and mechanical effects induced by dilation and hypertrophy,[31,32] have been proposed as possible mechanisms. Clinical and research data indicate that active and passive changes in the mechanical environment of the heart are capable of influencing the initiation and spread of cardiac excitation through pathways that are intrinsic to the heart, a phenomenon known as "mechanoelectric feedback."[33] One unifying explanation for the controversy about autonomic versus nonautonomic determinants of electrophysiologic adaptations in athletes could be that short-term physical training programs, such as those used in prospective studies, could induce autonomic adaptations, with a reduction in sympathetic activity and an increase in parasympathetic activity. Long-term aerobic training, accompanied by such anatomic changes as atrial and ventricular dilation, would create the mechanoelectric feedback necessary to induce intrinsic electrophysiologic adaptations, as demonstrated in cross-sectional studies.[29,31,32] Additionally, the loss of resting bradycardia that is seen with detraining, when studied in animal models, is associated with intrinsic heart changes that would, at least in part, explain these findings.[34]

Animals denervated before training did not develop intrinsic and rest bradycardia.[12] Thus, it is likely that a functioning autonomic system is necessary for the development of electrophysiologic adaptation.

OBSERVATIONAL STUDIES

It is well established that regularly exercising subjects have lower heart rates compared with sedentary subjects of the same age. Some classical observational studies,[35–37] using 24-hour ambulatory ECG monitoring, demonstrated that minimum, medium, and maximum heart rates of young high-level athletes (cyclists, long-distance runners, skiers, basketball players) were significantly lower compared with control subjects.

These changes are more commonly described in endurance athletes, as long-distance runners and cyclists (cyclic sports), not occurring frequently in power-training athletes. However, Balady and colleagues[38] have found similar results analyzing the ECGs of 289 professional football players (acyclic sport). The mean resting heart rate was 56 beats per minute (bpm), with 77% of the American football players having less than 60 bpm. Sinus arrhythmia was present in 7% and 24% had first-degree AV block. Morganroth and colleagues[39] also found bradycardia at rest in their population of wrestlers, who are also predominantly power-trained.

There is a different electrocardiography finding that can be seen in training athletes with a low heart rate (**Box 1**).

SINUS BRADYCARDIA AND SINUS ARRYTHMIAS

Sinus bradycardia and sinus arrhythmias are under the most common alterations found in the endurance athlete (**Fig. 1**). Sinus bradycardia is usually correlated to type and intensity of training.[6,9] Its incidence varies widely among the populations oscillating from 4% to 8% in general, to 40% to 90% in selected athlete's population.[40]

Box 1
ECG findings associated with low heart rate in athletes

Very Common
- Sinus bradycardia
- Sinus arrhythmia
- Sinus pauses

Common
- Wandering atrial pacemaker
- Junctional escape beats
- First-degree AV block
- Type I second-degree AV block (Wenckebach phenomenon)

Uncommon
- Type II second-degree AV block
- Third-degree AV block
- Sinoatrial type I block
- Sinoatrial exit block
- Ventricular escape beats

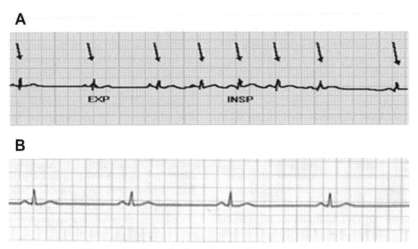

Fig. 1. (*A*) Sinus arrhythmia. (*B*) Sinus bradycardia, less than 40 bpm.

Sinus rates in the 30 to 40 bpm range are fairly common in the highly conditioned athlete.[41–43] The average of heart rate values in studies with high-level endurance athletes ranges between 53 and 10 bpm, showing that even in sports with high dynamic component the sinus bradycardia is not so low.[44] In cases of significant sinus bradycardia, a junctional or ventricular rhythm can compete with sinus rhythm. Typical isorhythmic dissociation is then observed. In a revision of 1964 high-level athletes' ECGs, just one case of idioventricular escape rhythm was found in a long-distance juvenile athlete.[45]

Associated with a slow sinus rate is respiratory sinus arrhythmia, which is the rhythmic change in heart rate with respiration. Sinus arrhythmia is mediated by atrial stretch receptors, which respond to increased and decreased venous return during inspiration and expiration by speeding or slowing heart rate, respectively. A more pronounced sinus bradycardia typically results in a more pronounced sinus arrhythmia. Junctional escape beats are not uncommon in athletes with slow sinus rates.[41] In up to 15% to 20% of athletes with sinus bradycardia can be found sinus arrhythmia, respiratory type in the youngsters, and in most of the cases not belonging to any type of sinoatrial block.[46] In Holter registry of 169 athletes, sinoatrial first-degree block was found in 10% of subjects, none of them presenting these findings on resting surface ECG.[47] Right atrium wandering atrial pacemakers are a frequent finding, ranging from 13.5% to 69% in trained individuals and present in up to 20% in the general population.[9]

Sharma and colleagues[48] performed an observational study with 1000 highly trained junior elite athletes and 300 nonathletic control subjects matched for gender, age, and body surface area. Athletes had a significantly higher prevalence of sinus bradycardia and sinus arrhythmia than nonathletes. Five percent of the athletes had first-degree AV block, 2% had nodal bradycardia, 1% had wandering atrial pacemaker, and another 1% had Mobitz type 1 second-degree AV block.

Sinus pauses are considerably frequent among athletes, with almost one-third of subjects presenting pauses superior to 2 seconds.[9] Viitasalo and colleagues[43] have found an incidence of 37% of sinus pauses in an athlete's sample.

AV CONDUCTION DISTURBANCES

Even if the PR interval can be augmented with vagal tone increasing, the occurrence of AV blocks depends mostly on individual susceptibility. The incidence of first- and second-degree AV block recorded by Holter in the classical studies of Palatini and coworkers, Talan and coworkers, and Viitasalo and coworkers[35–37] ranges from 27.5% to 40% for the first-degree and from 15% to 22% for the type I second-degree in athletes. Control groups incidence of first-degree AV block ranged from 5% to 14%, and type I second-degree ranged from 2.5% to 6%. None of these three studies found athletes with third-degree AV block.[35–37]

Zehender and colleagues[9] have found an incidence for first-degree AV block in 10% to 33% of observed athletes and approximately the same number had borderline PR values.[49] It is interesting to mention that under stress these individuals had shown a normalization of the PR interval.[49,50] Nakamato[50] observed second-degree type I AV block in 10% of marathon runners, which was clearly dependent on training conditions and occurred only at rest. Meytes and colleagues[51] found that the electrocardiographic incidence of this phenomenon in endurance athletes was only 2.4%. When long-term ECG follow-up was performed, the prevalence increased, ranging from 23% to 40%.[36,51] According to the same investigators the incidence of second-degree Mobitz 2 AV block in endurance athletes ranged from 2% to 8%.[37,52] The general incidence of third-degree AV block is 0.017% in athletes, being 100-fold that of the general population.[37,53] Of the total of 12,000 athletes evaluated by Fenici and colleagues,[53] five presented with a type II second-degree AV block and two with third-degree AV block. AV conduction normalized in all of these athletes with aerobic exercise. Zeppilli and colleagues[54] were able to revert these changes with Valsalva maneuver, exercise, and administration of atropine. In a Spanish study enrolling 3519 high-level athletes,[6] there was no case of high-grade ventricular blocks, depicting its lower incidence among trained subjects.

The bradyarrhythmias caused by increased vagal tone are usually physiologic, are favored by continued training, and are mostly asymptomatic.[35,55] They can be reverted with atropine use, hyperventilation, and exercise, and frequently disappear or decreased with detraining.

LONG-TERM FOLLOW-UP OF BRADYARRHYTHMIAS

A longitudinal follow-up study was performed in 157 former elite athletes, all of them with records of bradycardia (<50 bpm) when they were participating in high-level competition.[56] All had retired from competitive sport for a minimum of 5 years before participation in the follow-up examination. In the postretirement period, a total of 65% of participants had persistent bradycardia (18% with bradycardia <50 bpm). Multivariate analysis showed that persistence of resting bradycardia was associated with regular exercise and number of years in high-level training, but not with such symptoms as palpitations, dizziness, or syncope, or major ECG alterations.

Under 24-hour Holter monitoring, male veteran long-distance runners presented heart rates as low as 35 bpm, with nocturnal episodes of extreme bradycardia.[57] Interestingly, in older athletes, pathologic pauses and variable grade AV blocks are more frequent, maintaining a circadian variation and disappearing with exercise as in younger subjects. These differences are attributable to sinus and AV node dysfunction, secondary to aging and favored by training.

Box 2
ESC recommendations for interpretation of 12-lead ECG in the athlete with sinus bradycardia/arrhythmia

1. Only profound sinus bradycardia and/or marked sinus arrhythmia (heart rate less than 30 bpm and/or pauses ≥3 s during wake hours) need to be distinguished from sinus node disease.

2. Sino-atrial node dysfunction can be reasonably excluded by demonstrating that:

   a. Symptoms such as dizziness or syncope are absent

   b. Heart rate normalizes during exercise, sympathetic maneuvers or drugs, with preservation of maximal heart rate

   c. Bradycardia reverses with training reduction or discontinuation

From Corrado D, Pelliccia A, Heidbuchel H, et al. Recommendations for interpretation of 12-lead electrocardiogram in the athlete. Eur Heart J 2009;31:243–59; with permission.

In the long-term follow-up of former professional Swiss cyclists, sinus node disease, defined as bradycardia less than 40 bpm, atrial flutter, pacemaker need for the bradyarrhythmia, or maximal RR interval greater than 2.5 seconds were more common (16%) compared with healthy control subjects (2%).[58]

RECOMMENDATIONS

In 2009, an international group of experts under the auspices of the European Society of Cardiology (ESC) published new recommendations for

---

Box 3
ESC recommendations for interpretation of 12-lead ECG in the athlete with AV block

- Resolution of asymptomatic first or second-degree AV block with hyperventilation or exercise confirms its functional origin and excludes any pathologic significance.

- In athletes with Type II second-degree (Mobitz Type II) and third-degree AV block, a careful diagnostic evaluation is mandatory and pacemaker may be indicated.

From Corrado D, Pelliccia A, Heidbuchel H, et al. Recommendations for interpretation of 12-lead electrocardiogram in the athlete. Eur Heart J 2009;31:243–59; with permission.

the interpretation of the ECG in athletes.[59] Two years later, a consensus opinion of experts from many countries with decades of experience in dealing with athletes and ECGs was also published.[60] According to these seminal publications, sinus bradycardia, prolonged PR interval, and Wenckebach phenomenon are common in athletes as a result of the high resting vagal tone, or significantly lower intrinsic heart rates. As pointed out in both documents, there is no need to further evaluate sinus bradycardia as low as 30 bpm (with or without sinus arrhythmia). Prolonged PR interval up to 300 milliseconds should not prompt further work-up, but longer intervals should be resolved with an exercise test (the PR interval should shorten as vagal tone is withdrawn). Similarly, Wenckebach phenomenon in isolation need not prompt further work-up, but an exercise test could resolve any concern (the recommendations are summarized in **Boxes 2–4**).

REFERENCES

1. Blake JB, Larrabee RC. Observations upon long distance runners. Boston Med Surg J 1903;148:195.
2. Roeske WR, O'Rourke RA, Klein A. Noninvasive evaluation of ventricular hypertrophy in professional athletes. Circulation 1976;53:286–92.
3. Barach JH. Physiological and pathological effects of severe exertion (the marathon race) on the circulatory and renal systems. Arch Intern Med 1910;5:382.
4. Gordon B, Levine SA, Wilmaers A. Observations on a group of marathon runners. Arch Intern Med 1924;33:425.
5. Lichtman J, O'Rourke RA, Klein A, et al. Electrocardiogram of the athlete. Arch Intern Med 1973;32:763.
6. Perez AB, Fernandez LS. El corazón del deportista: hallazgos electrocardiográficos más frecuentes. Rev Esp Cardiol 1998;51:356–68.
7. Chapman JH. Profound sinus bradycardia in the athletic heart syndrome. J Sports Med Phys Fitness 1982;22:45–8.
8. Hanne-Paparo N, Kellermann JJ. Long-term Holter ECG monitoring of athletes. Med Sci Sports Exerc 1981;13:294–8.
9. Zehender M, Meinertz T, Keul J, et al. ECG variants and cardiac arrhythmia in athletes: clinical relevance and prognostic importance. Am Heart J 1990;119:1378–91.
10. Hammond HK, Froelicher VF. Normal and abnormal heart rate responses to exercise. Prog Cardiovasc Dis 1985;27:271–96.
11. Longhurst JC. Arterial baroreceptors in health and disease. Cardiovasc Rev Rep 1982;3:271–99.
12. Sigvardsson K, Svanfeldt E, Kilbom A. Role of the adrenergic nervous system in development of training induced bradycardia. Acta Physiol Scand 1977;101:481–8.
13. Clausen JP, Trap-Jensen J, Lassen NA. The effects of training on the heart rate during arm and leg exercise. Scand J Clin Lab Invest 1970;26:295–301.
14. Clausen JP, Klausen K, Rasmussen B, et al. Central and peripheral circulatory changes after training of the arms and legs. Am J Physiol 1973;225:675–82.
15. Smith ML, Hudson D, Graitzer H, et al. Exercise training bradycardia: the role of autonomic balance. Med Sci Sports Exerc 1989;21:40–8.
16. Yamamoto K, Miyachi M, Saitoh T, et al. Effects of endurance training on resting and post-exercise cardiac autonomic control. Med Sci Sports Exerc 2001;33:1496–502.
17. Carter JB, Banister EW, Blaber AP. Effect of endurance exercise on autonomic control of heart rate. Sports Med 2003;33:33–46.
18. Goldsmith RL, Bloomfeld DM, Rosenwinkel ET. Exercise and autonomic function. Coron Artery Dis 2000;11:129–35.
19. Areskog N. Effects and adverse effects of autonomic blockade in physical exercise. Am J Cardiol 1985;55:132–4.
20. Chen C, DiCarlo SE. Endurance exercise training-induces resting bradycardia: a brief review. Sports Med Train Rehabil 1997;8:37–77.
21. Wilmore JH, Stanforth P, Gagnon J, et al. Endurance exercise training has a minimal effect on resting heart rate: the HERITAGE study. Med Sci Sports Exerc 1996;28:829–35.
22. Shi X, Stevens G, Foresman B, et al. Autonomic nervous system control of the heart: endurance exercise training. Med Sci Sports Exerc 1995;27:1406–13.

23. Bouchard C, Rankinen T. Individual differences in response to regular physical activity. Med Sci Sports Exerc 2001;33:S446–51.

24. Blomqvist CG, Saltin S. Cardiovascular adaptations to physical training. Annu Rev Physiol 1983;45:169–89.

25. Smith SA, Querry RG, Fadel PJ, et al. Differential baroreflex control of heart rate in sedentary and aerobically fit individuals. Med Sci Sports Exerc 2000;32:1419–30.

26. Hughson RL, Yamamoto Y, Blaber AP, et al. Effect of 28- ay head down bed rest with counter measures on heart ate variability during LBNP. Aviat Space Environ Med 1994;65:293–300.

27. Sandercock GR, Bromley PD, Brodie DA. Effects of exercise on heart rate variability: inferences from meta-analysis. Med Sci Sports Exerc 2005;37:433–9.

28. Stein R, Moraes RS, Cavalcanti AV, et al. Atrial automaticity and atrioventricular conduction in athletes: contribution of autonomic regulation. Eur J Appl Physiol 2000;82:155–7.

29. Stein R, Medeiros CM, Rosito GA, et al. Intrinsic sinus and atrioventricular node electrophysiologic adaptations in endurance athletes. J Am Coll Cardiol 2002;39:1033–8.

30. Brorson L, Conradson TB, Olsson B, et al. Right atrial monophasic action potential and effective refractory periods in relation to physical training and maximal heart rate. Cardiovasc Res 1976;10:168–75.

31. Lewis SF, Nylander E, Gad P, et al. Non-autonomic component in bradycardia of endurance trained men at rest and during exercise. Acta Physiol Scand 1980;109:297–305.

32. Katona PG, McLean M, Dighton DH, et al. Sympathetic and parasympathetic cardiac control in athletes at rest. J Appl Physiol 1982;52:1652–7.

33. Kohl P, Hunter P, Noble D. Stretch-induced changes in heart rate and rhythm: clinical observations, experiments and mathematical models. Prog Biophys Mol Biol 1999;71:91–138.

34. Evangelista FS, Martuchi SE, Negrão CE, et al. Loss of resting bradycardia with detraining is associated with intrinsic heart rate changes control of heart rate with detraining Loss of resting bradycardia with detraining is associated with intrinsic heart rate changes. Braz J Med Biol Res 2005;38:1141–6.

35. Palatini P, Maraglino G, Sperti G, et al. Prevalence and possible mechanisms of ventricular arrhythmias in athletes. Am Heart J 1985;110:560–7.

36. Talan DA, Bauernfeind RA, Ashley WW, et al. Twenty-four hour continuous ECG recordings in long-distance runners. Chest 1982;82:19–24.

37. Viitasalo M, Kala R, Eisalo A. Ambulatory electrocardiographic recording in endurance athletes. Br Heart J 1982;47:213–20.

38. Balady GJ, Cadigan JB, Ryan TJ. Electrocardiogram of the athlete: an analysis of 289 professional football. Am J Cardiol 1984;53:1339–43.

39. Morganroth J, Yaron BJ, Henry WJ, et al. Comparative left ventricular dimensions in trained athletes. Ann Intern Med 1975;82:521–4.

40. Zeppilli P, Cecchetti F. L'elettrocardiogramma dell'atleta. In: Zeppilli P, editor. Cardiologia dello sport. Roma (Italy): CESI; 1996. p. 149.

41. Huston TP, Puffer JC, Rodney WM. The athletic heart syndrome. N Engl J Med 1985;313:24–32.

42. Wight JN Jr, Salem D. Sudden cardiac death and the athletic heart. Arch Intern Med 1995;155:1473–80.

43. Viitasalo MT, Kala R, Eisalo A. Ambulatory electrocardiographic findings in young athletes between 14 and 16 years of age. Eur Heart J 1984;5:2–6.

44. Douglas PS, O'Toole ML, Hiller DB, et al. Electrocardiographic diagnosis of exercise-induced left ventricular hypertrophy. Am Heart J 1988;116:784–90.

45. Boraita A. Arritmias cardiacas y su implicación con la actividad física. In: Ferrer López V, Martínez Riaza L, Santoja Medina F, editors. Escolar: medicina y deporte. Albacete (Spain): Diputación de Albacete; 1996. p. 98.

46. Venerando A. Electrocardiography in sports medicine. J Sports Med Phys Fitness 1979;19:107–28.

47. Boraita A, Serratosa L, Antón P, et al. Las arritmias del deportista. Rev Lat Cardiol 1996;17:124–31.

48. Sharma S, Whyte G, Elliott P, et al. Electrocardiographic changes in 1000 highly trained junior elite athletes. Br J Sports Med 1999;33:319–24.

49. Van Ganse W, Versee L, Eylenbosch W, et al. The electrocardiogram of athletes: comparison with untrained subjects. Br Heart J 1970;32:160–4.

50. Nakamoto K. Electrocardiograms of 25 marathon runners before and after 100 meter dash. Jpn Circ J 1969;33:105–28.

51. Meytes I, Kaplinsky E, Yahini JH. Wenckenbach A-V block: a frequent feature following heavy physical training. Am Heart J 1975;90:426–30.

52. Underwood RH, Schwade JL. Noninvasive analyses of cardiac function of elite distance runners: echocardiography, vectorcardiography, and cardiac intervals. Ann N Y Acad Sci 1977;301:297–309.

53. Fenici R, Caselli G, Seppilli P, et al. High degree A-V block in 17 well-trained endurance athletes. In: Lubich T, Venerando A, editors. Sports cardiology. Bologna (Italy): Aulo Gaggi; 1980. p. 523–37.

54. Zeppilli P, Fenici R, Sassara M, et al. Wenckenbach secon-degree AV block in top-ranking athletes: an old problem revisited. Am Heart J 1980;100:291–4.

55. Pantano JA, Oriel RJ. Prevalence and nature of cardiac arrhythmias in apparently normal well trained runners. Am Heart J 1982;104:762–8.

56. Serra-Grima R, Puig T, Doñate M, et al. Long-term follow-up of bradycardia in elite athletes. Int J Sports Med 2008;29:934–7.

57. Northcote RJ, Canning GP, Ballantyne D. Electrocardiographic findings in male veteran endurance athletes. Br Heart J 1989;61:155–60.

58. Baldesberger S, Bauersfeld U, Candinas R, et al. Sinus node disease and arrhythmias in the long-term follow-up of former professional cyclists. Eur Heart J 2008;29:71–8.

59. Corrado D, Pelliccia A, Heidbuchel H, et al. Recommendations for Interpretation of 12-lead electrocardiogram in the athlete. Eur Heart J 2009;31:243–59.

60. Uberoi A, Stein R, Perez VM, et al. Interpretation of the electrocardiogram of young athletes. Circulation 2011;124:746–57.

Prevalence and Management of Atrial Fibrillation in Middle-Aged/Older Athletes

Stefania Sacchi, MD[a], Giuseppe Mascia, MD[a],
Luigi Di Biase, MD, PhD[b,c,d,i], Pasquale Santangeli, MD[b,d],
John David Burkhardt, MD[b], Luigi Padeletti, MD[a],
Andrea Natale, MD[b,c,e,f,g,h],*

KEYWORDS

- Atrial fibrillation • Ablation • Athletes • Inflammatory response

KEY POINTS

- Atrial fibrillation (AF) in middle-aged/older athletes has a low prevalence.
- Sports activity may represent a facilitating factor anticipating the AF onset, but does not represent the cause of AF.
- AF ablation represents a valid therapeutic option in these subjects.

INTRODUCTION

Atrial fibrillation (AF) is the most common arrhythmia in clinical practice.[1] The estimated prevalence of AF is 0.4% to 1% in the general population, increasing with age to 8% in those older than 80 years.[2] AF is also the most common arrhythmia in the athletic community.[3] Recent data have documented a relationship between endurance sport practice and risk of AF, but reports from epidemiologic studies demonstrating AF in athletes have been variable because of the study population's age, years of training, and associated comorbidities.[4–12]

PREVALENCE AND INCIDENCE OF ATRIAL FIBRILLATION IN ATHLETES

The prevalence of AF in the athletic community ranges from 0.2% to 60% and AF is more frequently observed in middle-aged than in young athletes.[3] Furlanello and colleagues[13] reported that AF accounted for up to 0.2% in a population of 5000 athletes. Pelliccia and colleagues[14] reported that

Conflict of Interest: Dr Andrea Natale has received consultant fees or honoraria from Biosense Webster, Boston Scientific, Medtronic, Biotronik, and LifeWatch. Dr Luigi Di Biase has received consultant fees from Biosense Webster and Hansen Medical. Dr Luigi Padeletti is a consultant for Boston Scientific, Medtronic, St. Jude Medical, Biotronik, Sorin Biomedica. The other authors declare no conflicts of interest.

[a] Department of Heart and Vessels, University of Florence, Viale Morgagni 85, 50141 Florence, Italy; [b] Texas Cardiac Arrhythmia Institute, St. David's Medical Center, 3000 North I-35, Suite 720, Austin, TX 78705, USA; [c] Department of Biomedical Engineering, University of Texas, 107 W Dean Keeton Street Stop C0800, Austin, TX 78712, USA; [d] Department of Cardiology, University of Foggia, Viale Pinto 1, 71100 Foggia, Italy; [e] Division of Cardiology, Stanford University, Palo Alto, 300 Pasteur Dr MC 5319 A260 Stanford, CA 94305, USA; [f] EP section, Case Western Reserve University, Cleveland, OH, USA; [g] Interventional Electrophysiology, Scripps Clinic, 10666 N Torrey Pines Road, SW206 La Jolla, San Diego, CA 92037, USA; [h] EP and Arrhythmia Services, California Pacific Medical Center, 2333 Buchanan Street, San Francisco, CA 94115, USA; [i] Albert Einstein College of Medicine at Montefiore Hospital, Section of Electrophysiology, 1825 Eastchester Road, Bronx, NY 10461-2301, USA

* Corresponding author. Texas Cardiac Arrhythmia Institute, St. David's Medical Center, 3000 North I-35, Suite 720, Austin, TX 78705.
E-mail address: dr.natale@gmail.com

Card Electrophysiol Clin 5 (2013) 115–121
http://dx.doi.org/10.1016/j.ccep.2012.11.002

the prevalence of AF was 0.3% in a study involving 1776 subjects. It should be noted that they reported an incidence of lone AF among competitive athletes similar to that observed in the general population.[11] However, their studies were performed in young athletes, with relatively few years of training and at the moment of highest activity.

STUDIES DEMONSTRATING AN INCREASED RISK OF ATRIAL FIBRILLATION IN MIDDLE-AGED/OLDER ATHLETES

In contrast with these previous data, several other studies have shown an increased proportion of AF in athletes compared with the rest of the population and those supporting the association between long-term endurance sport practice and AF have been performed in middle-aged individuals, after many years of training.[11]

Karjalainen and colleagues[4] in 1998 were the first to publish a longitudinal prospective case-control study establishing a relationship between endurance sport practice and AF. They studied a series of orienteers, endurance cross-country runners. Mean age at baseline was 47.5 years in orienteers and 49.6 years in controls. After 10 years of follow-up, AF had been diagnosed in 12 of 228 (5.3%) orienteers and in 2 of 212 (0.9%) control subjects. The odds ratio for AF associated with vigorous exercise was 5.5. The authors concluded that vigorous long-term exercise was associated with AF in healthy middle-aged men despite protecting against coronary heart disease and premature death.[4]

Mont and colleagues[5] found that endurance sport practice was much more prevalent among patients with lone AF compared with the general population. The proportion of regular sport practice among middle-aged men with lone AF was much higher than among men from the general population (63% vs 15%). A rather lax definition of sport practice was used (more than 3 hours a week at the moment of evaluation), but most patients had been involved in endurance sport practice for more than 10 years, with much higher levels of participation in the past. These data suggested that chronic sport practice may contribute to the development of AF in male patients.[5]

The same population of lone AF patients was analyzed in a case-control study with 2 age-matched controls for each case from the general population (mean age, 41 ± 13 AF patients, 44 ± 11 controls).[6] The analysis showed that the current sport practice increased the risk of developing lone AF more than 5 times, a result that was within the range reported by Karjalainen and colleagues. It is noteworthy that the association of current sport

practice with lone AF was observed at more than 1500 lifetime hours of sport practice, suggesting the existence of a threshold point. Of course, this threshold point should be interpreted with caution.[6]

To confirm the association between endurance sports and AF in a longitudinal manner, Molina and colleagues[8] undertook a study that included 183 individuals (mean age, 39 ± 9 years) who ran the Barcelona Marathon in 1992 and 290 sedentary healthy individuals (mean age, 50 ± 13 years) included in the REGICOR study. After 10 years of follow-up, the annual incidence rate of lone AF among marathon runners and sedentary men was 0.43/100 and 0.11/100, respectively. Endurance sport practice was associated with a higher risk of incident lone AF in the multivariate age-adjusted and blood pressure–adjusted Cox regression models. The main limitation of this study was the small number of events observed during follow-up (n = 9 among marathon runners and n = 2 among sedentary men). Nevertheless, the results were consistent with previous observations.[8] Moreover, in a prospective study on high-performance male participants in endurance cross-country ski competitions after 28 to 30 years of follow-up, Grimsmo and colleagues[15] found an 18% prevalence of lone AF in athletes whose mean age was 58 years at follow-up. This prevalence was at least 10 times higher than expected in age-matched controls.[15]

Most of the described series include patients suffering concomitant AF and atrial flutter, suggesting that endurance sports contribute to the development of both arrhythmias.[11] Heidbüchel and colleagues[7] found that a history of endurance sports in middle-aged patients, defined as semi-competitive participation in cycling, running, or swimming for ≥3 h/week (and for ≥3 years preablation), was a significant risk factor for AF after common flutter ablation. Also, continuation of endurance sport activity after ablation showed a trend for increased risk of developing AF.[7]

Recently, Van Buuren and colleagues[16] studied 33 former top-level handball players from the first German league (57 ± 5 years). Data were compared with 24 sedentary healthy controls. Ten of 33 athletes suffered from AF. The authors demonstrated that not only endurance training but also sports activity with a relevant static component, like team handball, might predispose for AF over the age of 50. More data in nonendurance sports are mandatory to confirm this hypothesis.[16] All these studies seem to have established that long-lasting endurance sport practice increases the risk of lone AF in the middle-aged athletes. In addition, vigorous physical activity associated with occupational activities may pose a similar risk.[11] Data from the GIRAFA study seem to confirm this theory.[9] The prospective GIRAFA study was conducted in consecutive patients with lone AF recruited at the emergency room. In this case-control study, 107 lone AF patients (mean age, 48 ± 11 years) were compared with age-matched and sex-matched healthy controls. Total hours of physical activity (during work or leisure time) were collected with a detailed and validated questionnaire. For each physical activity, the following variables were recorded: age started, age ended, months per year, days per week, and hours per day. Subjects were asked to classify the intensity of each physical activity in 4 levels: sedentary, light, moderate, and heavy. The results showed that the moderate and heavy physical activity, whether sport-related or job-related, increased the risk of suffering AF.[9]

DOES SPORT PRACTICE ANTICIPATE THE ONSET OF ATRIAL FIBRILLATION?

Some studies showed that endurance sports activity might increase the risk of developing atrial fibrillation in healthy middle-aged men.[4–12] Molina and colleagues[8] found that the risk of AF in physically active subjects is associated with both a larger left atrial inferosuperior diameter and a larger left atrial volume. Mont and colleagues[9] found that anteroposterior atrial diameter was independently associated with lone AF in middle-aged healthy individuals. In addition, it has been shown that in athletes suffering from cardiac diseases, sports activity might facilitate both atrial and ventricular arrhythmias.[8,9,17] Delise and colleagues[18] nicely showed that this correlation (endurance sport activity and AF) is weak and arose from limited and unconvincing data. It is the authors' opinion, as well as reported by Delise and colleagues,[18] that AF is not the consequence of endurance sports in the athletes. The reported incidence is in fact less than 0.5% in healthy subjects without comorbidities. It could be speculated that endurance sports represent a facilitating factor anticipating the onset of AF that would have probably occurred anyway but at a later time in life. In individuals with cardiovascular disorders, the correlation arrhythmias/endurance sport activity cannot be excluded. However, the benefit/risk ratio of performing endurance sports to reducing risk factors versus facilitating arrhythmias onset favors the performance of sport activities.

PATHOPHYSIOLOGY OF EXERCISE-RELATED ATRIAL FIBRILLATION

Several mechanisms may be acting together in exercise-related AF. It is well accepted that arrhythmias depend on triggers, substrates, and modulators and that these factors may be present in relation to physical activity.[11] Atrial ectopy, particularly pulmonary vein ectopy, has been shown to be the trigger in most episodes of paroxysmal AF,[19] and atrial and ventricular ectopy may be increased as a consequence of physical activity.[20,21] Nevertheless, the hypothesis of increased atrial ectopy as an explanation for the association between sports and AF cannot be adequately sustained with currently available data.[11] There are some data suggesting that combined hyperactivation of parasympathetic and sympathetic systems in athletes can be proarrhythmic.[22] According to the GIRAFA study, vagal AF is a more common form of lone AF, demonstrating that 70% of consecutive patients with lone AF had vagal AF.[9] Experimental data also show that increased vagal tone shortens and increases the dispersion of the atrial refractory period, creating the conditions required for reentry.[23] Therefore, the increased vagal tone induced by sport practice may indeed facilitate the appearance of AF.[3]

Whether there is a structural substrate in lone AF is still a matter of debate. It is plausible that long-term endurance sport practice or occupational physical activity may induce structural changes in the atrium (enlargement, fibrosis) that may create a favorable substrate for the disease.[11] In fact, Frustaci and colleagues[24] found structural changes in a series of 12 patients with paroxysmal, recurrent, drug refractory lone AF. Trivax and McCullough recently proposed the term "Philippides cardiomyopathy" for the development of multiple cardiac abnormalities associated with endurance sports.[25] Vigorous exercise increases the demand for oxygen, release of catecholamines, and changes in free fatty acid metabolism, determining acute effects (dilatation, diastolic dysfunction), subacute effects (overexpression of cardiac fibrotic marker, collagens, and fibronectin-1), and finally, chronic effects, developing areas of fibrosis, a substrate for both AF and ventricular arrhythmias.[25] The role of fibrosis has also been evaluated in experimental models.[26,27]

Among older adults, the pathophysiology of AF may be different and often related to increased vascular stiffness and reduced left ventricular compliance, as reflected by risk factors for AF, such as higher systolic blood pressure, treated hypertension, prior myocardial infarction, congestive heart failure, valvular heart disease, and left atrial enlargement. Based on these risk factors in older adults, habitual physical activity might be expected to reduce the incidence of AF, for example, by reducing blood pressure, improving vascular compliance, or reducing risk of myocardial infarction or congestive heart failure.[28]

The Cardiovascular Health Study prospectively investigated the association of leisure-time activity, exercise intensity, and walking habits with the incidence of AF in older adults. Mozaffarian and colleagues[28] found that greater leisure-time activity and walking were associated with graded lower incidence of AF, with progressively lower risk as both leisure-time activity and distances and paces of walking increased. Conversely, intensity of exercise had a U-shaped relationship with AF, with lower risk among individuals exercising with moderate, but not high intensity. In contrast to prior retrospective reports and case series, high-intensity exercise was not associated with higher AF risk; this could relate to relatively lower maximal intensity of exercise in these older adults compared with younger adults or to different pathoetiology of AF later in life.[28] However, high-intensity exercise was also not associated with lower AF risk, suggesting an overall net neutral association of high-intensity exercise with AF incidence in older adults. In comparison, moderate physical activities, such as greater leisure-time activity, distances and paces of walking, and moderate intensity exercise, were associated with significantly lower risk.

These results suggested that long-term benefits for AF risk of light or moderate physical activities in older adults outweigh any potential higher risk of AF associated with the acute activity or exercise.[28] Another factor that has been involved in the genesis of AF is the use of anabolic steroids.[29,30] Although some isolated case reports show a link between AF and steroids, the cases have presented in young athletes, at the moment of maximal physical activity, whereas AF in endurance sports seems to occur in middle-aged men, years after cessation of professional competitive or maximal activity. Therefore, although anabolic steroids may have a role in the genesis of AF, it is probably marginal.[11]

RELATIONSHIP BETWEEN ENDURANCE SPORT PRACTICE AND INFLAMMATORY RESPONSE

The skeletal muscle has been recently identified as an endocrine organ[31] and it has been suggested that cytokines that are released by muscle fibers determining paracrine, autocrine, and endocrine effects should be classified as myokines.[32] Recently, Vella and colleagues[33] proposed that intense exercise activates NF-κB signaling, a key transcription factor in the regulation of myokines mediating the postexercise inflammation, in skeletal muscle. Recent review of the literature by Swanson[34] shows a relationship between AF and C-reactive protein; moreover, Kasapis and Thompson[35] described a connection between interleukin-6 (IL-6) plasma concentration and endurance exercise, confirming that excessive endurance exercise can lead to chronic system inflammation. In addition, many authors found an association between C-reactive protein, IL-6, and both the presence of AF and the risk of developing future AF.[36–38] Chung and colleagues[36] studied 131 patients with atrial arrhythmia and 71 control patients and found C-reactive protein elevation in AF patients. Elevation of C-reactive protein was greatest in patients with more persistent AF. Psychari and colleagues[37] enrolled 90 patients with AF (persistent and permanent) and 46 control patients and found that both C-reactive protein and IL-6 participate in the evolution of AF and correlate with left atrium size. Therefore, the increase of C-reactive protein and IL-6 was related to anatomic changes and both were positively related to the diameter of the left atrium.[37] Malouf and colleagues[38] studied 67 patients with AF or atrial flutter who underwent successful electrical cardioversion (CV) and found that the C-reactive protein was predictive of an increased risk of recurrence of arrhythmias within 1 month after successful electrical cardioversion (**Fig. 1**).

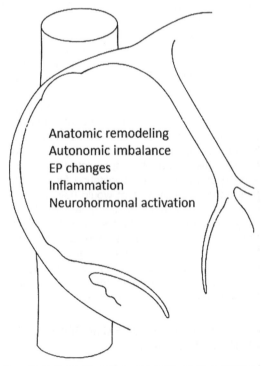

Anatomic remodeling
Autonomic imbalance
EP changes
Inflammation
Neurohormonal activation

Fig. 1. Factors favoring atrial fibrillation (AF) in athletes. EP, electrophysiologic.

MANAGEMENT OF ATRIAL FIBRILLATION IN ATHLETES

With regard to the AF treatment in athletes, the most important aspect is recognizing cases as a manifestation of "overtraining syndrome."[3] In such cases, it may be prudent to interrupt sports training and control of AF recurrence. Furlanello and colleagues[13] described a good response to sports abstinence in 1772 top-level athletes with AF. However, there are few data that the limitation of sports activities can have favorable outcomes in athletes with AF. In addition to this, treatment of AF in athletes is similar to other patient populations with obvious limitations.[3] β-Blockers may not be of much use in athletes, not only because they may reduce sports performance but also because β-blockers are prohibited in competition in specific sports, reported in the World Anti-Doping Agency list.[39] Other rate-control medications, such as calcium channel blockers and digoxin, have limited use for similar reasons.[3] There is a potential role of angiotensin-converting enzyme inhibitors and angiotensin receptor blockers in preventing AF recurrence, especially after ablation.[40,41] Antiarrhythmic drugs are typically quite effective in individuals without heart disease; type IC agents, such as flecainide or propafenone, are generally preferred as initial agents because of the safety profile and efficacy of these drugs. The use of amiodarone is not advised because of the long-term side effects and impairment of quality of life; dronedarone has yet to prove its efficacy in athletes but, considering its rate-slowing effect, it may not be as useful in this group of patients because it may impair sports performance.[3,42] Regardless of the rate versus rhythm control strategy, the need for anticoagulation is based on stroke risk factors. Long-term anticoagulation with a vitamin K antagonist, a direct thrombin inhibitor, or a factor Xa inhibitor is not recommended for primary prevention of stroke in patients with lone AF without any risk factors for thromboembolism, especially in athletes in whom the risk for bleeding is high.[3] Therefore the value of ablation in lone AF is emerging and there are some data proving its efficacy in athletes.[43] Furlanello and colleagues[44] investigated the effectiveness of catheter ablation of idiopathic drug-refractory AF in 20 athletes with palpitations depressing physical performance and compromising eligibility for competitive activities. Eighteen patients (90%) were free of AF and 2 (10%) reported short-lasting (minutes) episodes of palpitations during a mean follow-up of 3 years. Moreover, at follow-up, all baseline quality-of-life parameters pertinent to physical activity significantly improved, and all athletes obtained re-eligibility and could effectively reinitiate sport activity. In the study of Calvo and colleagues,[45] circumferential pulmonary vein ablation was effective in both endurance sport AF and other AF causes. Calvo and colleagues proved that the probability of remaining free of AF recurrences after a single circumferential pulmonary vein ablation was similar in athletes compared with the rest of the population after a mean follow-up of 18.69 ± 11.7 months. Also, Koopman and colleagues[46] showed that in patients with documented focal induction of nonpermanent AF and absence of structural heart disease, pulmonary vein isolation (PVI) was as effective in endurance athletes as in other patients. On the other hand, Heidbüchel and colleagues[7] found an increased incidence of AF after successful flutter ablation among endurance athletes.

SUMMARY

There is no evidence supporting the hypothesis that endurance sport activity is the cause of AF in healthy middle-aged athletes. Endurance sports in these subjects may facilitate or anticipate the AF onset, which would have occurred anyway at a later time in life. Catheter ablation of AF is an attractive option for athletes (especially young), who have a normal heart, and face a lifetime of AF risk.[47] However, randomized clinical trials with a larger number of patients are necessary to further understand if endurance sport practice plays an important role on the maintenance of stable sinus rhythm following catheter ablation of AF.

REFERENCES

1. Go AS, Hylek EM, Phillips KA, et al. Prevalence of diagnosed atrial fibrillation in adults: national implications for rhythm management and stroke prevention: the AnTicoagulation and Risk Factors in Atrial Fibrillation (ATRIA) Study. JAMA 2001; 285(18):2370–5.
2. Furberg CD, Psaty BM, Manolio TA, et al. Prevalence of atrial fibrillation in elderly subjects (the Cardiovascular Health Study). Am J Cardiol 1994;74(3): 236–41.
3. Turagam MK, Velagapudi P, Kocheril AG. Atrial fibrillation in athletes. Am J Cardiol 2012;109(2): 296–302.
4. Karjalainen J, Kujala UM, Kaprio J, et al. Lone atrial fibrillation in vigorously exercising middle aged men: case-control study. BMJ 1998;316(7147):1784–5.
5. Mont L, Sambola A, Brugada J, et al. Long-lasting sport practice and lone atrial fibrillation. Eur Heart J 2002;23(6):477–8.

6. Elosua R, Arquer A, Mont L, et al. Sport practice and the risk of lone atrial fibrillation: a case-control study. Int J Cardiol 2006;108(3):332–7.

7. Heidbüchel H, Anné W, Willems R, et al. Endurance sports is a risk factor for atrial fibrillation after ablation for atrial flutter. Int J Cardiol 2006;107(1):67–72.

8. Molina L, Mont L, Marrugat J, et al. Long-term endurance sport practice increases the incidence of lone atrial fibrillation in men: a follow-up study. Europace 2008;10(5):612–23.

9. Mont L, Tamborero D, Elosua R, et al. GIRAFA (Grup Integrat de Recerca en Fibril-lació Auricular) Investigators. Physical activity, height, and left atrial size are independent risk factors for lone atrial fibrillation in middle-aged healthy individuals. Europace 2008; 10(1):15–20.

10. Taggar JS, Lip GY. Risk predictors for lone atrial fibrillation. Europace 2008;10(1):6–8.

11. Mont L, Elosua R, Brugada J. Endurance sport practice as a risk factor for atrial fibrillation and atrial flutter. Europace 2009;11(1):11–7.

12. Abdulla J, Nielsen JR. Is the risk of atrial fibrillation higher in athletes than in the general population? A systematic review and meta-analysis. Europace 2009;11(9):1156–9.

13. Furlanello F, Bertoldi A, Dallago M, et al. Atrial fibrillation in elite athletes. J Cardiovasc Electrophysiol 1998;9(Suppl 8):S63–8.

14. Pelliccia A, Maron BJ, Di Paolo FM, et al. Prevalence and clinical significance of left atrial remodeling in competitive athletes. J Am Coll Cardiol 2005;46(4): 690–6.

15. Grimsmo J, Grundvold I, Maehlum S, et al. High prevalence of atrial fibrillation in long-term endurance cross-country skiers: echocardiographic findings and possible predictors–a 28–30 years follow-up study. Eur J Cardiovasc Prev Rehabil 2010;17(1):100–5.

16. Van Buuren F, Mellwig KP, Faber L, et al. The occurrence of atrial fibrillation in former top-level handball players above the age of 50. Acta Cardiol 2012; 67(2):213–20.

17. Corrado D, Basso C, Rizzoli G, et al. Does sports activity enhance the risk of sudden death in adolescents and young adults? J Am Coll Cardiol 2003;42: 1959–63.

18. Delise P, Sitta N, Berton G. Does long-lasting sports practice increase the risk of atrial fibrillation in healthy middle-aged men? Weak suggestions, no objective evidence. J Cardiovasc Med (Hagerstown) 2012;13(6):381–5.

19. Haïssaguerre M, Jaïs P, Shah DC, et al. Spontaneous initiation of atrial fibrillation by ectopic beats originating in the pulmonary veins. N Engl J Med 1998;339(10):659–66.

20. Baldesberger S, Bauersfeld U, Candinas R, et al. Sinus node disease and arrhythmias in the long-term follow-up of former professional cyclists. Eur Heart J 2008;29(1):71–8.

21. Bjørnstad H, Storstein L, Meen HD, et al. Ambulatory electrocardiographic findings in top athletes, athletic students and control subjects. Cardiology 1994;84(1):42–50.

22. Sharifov OF, Fedorov VV, Beloshapko GG, et al. Roles of adrenergic and cholinergic stimulation in spontaneous atrial fibrillation in dogs. J Am Coll Cardiol 2004;43(3):483–90.

23. Moe GK, Abildskov JA. Atrial fibrillation as a self-sustaining arrhythmia independent of focal discharge. Am Heart J 1959;58(1):59–70.

24. Frustaci A, Chimenti C, Bellocci F, et al. Histological substrate of atrial biopsies in patients with lone atrial fibrillation. Circulation 1997;96(4):1180–4.

25. Trivax JE, McCullough PA. Phidippides cardiomyopathy: a review and case illustration. Clin Cardiol 2012;35(2):69–73.

26. Benito B, Gay-Jordi G, Serrano-Mollar A, et al. Cardiac arrhythmogenic remodeling in a rat model of long-term intensive exercise training. Circulation 2011;123(1):13 22.

27. Lachance D, Plante E, Bouchard-Thomassin AA, et al. Moderate exercise training improves survival and ventricular remodeling in an animal model of left ventricular volume overload. Circ Heart Fail 2009;2(5):437–45.

28. Mozaffarian D, Furberg CD, Psaty BM, et al. Physical activity and incidence of atrial fibrillation in older adults: the cardiovascular health study. Circulation 2008;118(8):800–7.

29. Sullivan ML, Martinez CM, Gallagher EJ. Atrial fibrillation and anabolic steroids. J Emerg Med 1999; 17(5):851–7.

30. Lau DH, Stiles MK, John B, et al. Atrial fibrillation and anabolic steroid abuse. Int J Cardiol 2007;117(2): e86–7.

31. Pedersen BK, Febbraio MA. Muscle as an endocrine organ: focus on muscle-derived interleukin-6. Physiol Rev 2008;88:1379–406.

32. Febbraio MA, Pedersen BK. Contraction-induced myokine production and release: is skeletal muscle an endocrine organ? Exerc Sport Sci Rev 2005;33: 114–9.

33. Vella L, Caldow MK, Larsen AE, et al. Resistance exercise increases NF-κB activity in human skeletal muscle. Am J Physiol 2012;302:R667–73.

34. Swanson DR. Atrial fibrillation in athletes: implicit literature-based connections suggest that overtraining and subsequent inflammation may be a contributory mechanism. Med Hypotheses 2006; 66(6):1085–92.

35. Kasapis C, Thompson PD. The effects of physical activity on serum C-reactive protein and inflammatory markers: a systematic review. J Am Coll Cardiol 2005;45(10):1563–9.

36. Chung MK, Martin DO, Sprecher D, et al. C-reactive protein elevation in patients with atrial arrhythmias: inflammatory mechanisms and persistence of atrial fibrillation. Circulation 2001;104:2886–91.

37. Psychari SN, Apostolou TS, Sinos L, et al. Relation of elevated C-reactive protein and interleukin-6 levels to left atrial size and duration of episodes in patients with atrial fibrillation. Am J Cardiol 2005;95(6):764–7.

38. Malouf JF, Kanagala R, Al Atawi FO, et al. High-sensitivity C-reactive protein. A novel predictor for recurrence of atrial fibrillation after successful cardioversion. J Am Coll Cardiol 2005;46:1284–7.

39. World Anti-Doping Agency. Home page. Available at: http://www.wada-ama.org/en/World-Anti-Doping-Program/Sports-and-Anti-Doping-Organizations/International-Standards/Prohibited-List/. Accessed March 27, 2012.

40. Annè W, Willems R, Van der Merwe N, et al. Atrial fibrillation after radiofrequency ablation of atrial flutter: preventive effect of angiotensin converting enzyme inhibitors, angiotensin II receptor blockers, and diuretics. Heart 2004;90(9):1025–30.

41. Madrid AH, Bueno MG, Rebollo JM, et al. Use of irbesartan to maintain sinus rhythm in patients with long-lasting persistent atrial fibrillation: a prospective and randomized study. Circulation 2002;106(3):331–6.

42. Link MS, Estes NA. Athletes and arrhythmias. J Cardiovasc Electrophysiol 2010;21(10):1184–9.

43. Fuster V, Rydén LE, Cannom DS, et al, American College of Cardiology, American Heart Association Task Force, European Society of Cardiology Committee for Practice Guidelines, European Heart Rhythm Association, Heart Rhythm Society. ACC/AHA/ESC 2006 guidelines for the management of patients with atrial fibrillation: full text: a report of the American College of Cardiology/American Heart Association Task Force on practice guidelines and the European Society of Cardiology Committee for Practice Guidelines (Writing Committee to Revise the 2001 guidelines for the management of patients with atrial fibrillation) developed in collaboration with the European Heart Rhythm Association and the Heart Rhythm Society. Europace 2006;8(9):651–745.

44. Furlanello F, Lupo P, Pittalis M, et al. Radiofrequency catheter ablation of atrial fibrillation in athletes referred for disabling symptoms preventing usual training schedule and sport competition. J Cardiovasc Electrophysiol 2008;19(5):457–62.

45. Calvo N, Mont L, Tamborero D, et al. Efficacy of circumferential pulmonary vein ablation of atrial fibrillation in endurance athletes. Europace 2010;12(1):30–6.

46. Koopman P, Nuyens D, Garweg C, et al. Efficacy of radiofrequency catheter ablation in athletes with atrial fibrillation. Europace 2011;13(10):1386–93.

47. Mascia G, Perrotta L, Galanti G, et al. Atrial fibrillation in athletes. Int J Sports Med 2012. [Epub ahead of print].

Implantable Cardioverter-Defibrillator Therapy in Athletes

Mohamed ElMaghawry, MD[a,b], Federico Migliore, MD[a],
Alessandro Zorzi, MD[a], Barbara Bauce, MD, PhD[a],
Loira Leoni, MD, PhD[a], Emanuele Bertaglia, MD[a],
Sabino Iliceto, MD[a], Domenico Corrado, MD, PhD[a,*]

KEYWORDS

- Athlete • Implantable cardioverter-defibrillator • Sudden cardiac death • Arrhythmia

KEY POINTS

- There are few data assessing the benefits and risks of sports participation for patients with implantable cardioverter-defibrillators (ICDs).
- Sports may affect the performance of an ICD with the potential for failure of therapy, inappropriate interventions, and damage to the device system.
- Sports may have a hazardous effect on the natural history of many cardiovascular diseases.
- Despite some controversies, current recommendations restrict competitive sports participation in patients with ICDs.

INTRODUCTION

Since the implantable cardioverter-defibrillator (ICD) was first used in humans in 1980,[1] major developments have been witnessed in the technological, diagnostic, and therapeutic aspects of this life-saving modality. Many seminal multicenter trials have helped to broaden the range of indications for ICD implantation for primary and secondary prevention of sudden cardiac death (SCD) to include not only ischemic heart failure but also various types of cardiomyopathies and cardiac ion channelopathies.[2–11] The exponential increase in the rates of ICD implantations has been accompanied with the emergence of some clinical problems and dilemmas that physicians dealing with ICDs may face. Management of athletes with ICDs represents one of these challenges. Regular physical exercise has been established to lower cardiovascular risk[12,13] and improve quality of life[14]; however, sports activity is associated with an increased risk of SCD because of malignant ventricular arrhythmias in susceptible athletes with cardiovascular diseases.[15] ICD therapy would offer protection against arrhythmic events in this subgroup of athletes. However, ICD performance may be affected by sports activity, with the potential risk of failure of therapy, inappropriate interventions, and device injury. American and European recommendations do not allow most competitive sports in patients carrying ICDs.[16,17] On the other hand, some recent studies have raised concerns on such restrictive recommendations by proving the safety of ICD therapy

Disclosures: No conflicts of interest to declare.
Sources of funding: This study was supported by Fondazione Cariparo, Padova and Rovigo, Italy; and Registry of Cardio-Cerebro-Vascular Pathology, Veneto Region, Venice, Italy.
[a] Division of Cardiology, Department of Cardiac, Thoracic and Vascular Sciences, University of Padova, Via Giustiniani 2, 35120, Padova, Italy; [b] Department of Cardiology, Aswan Heart Centre, Kasr El Hajjar Street, PO Box 81512, Aswan, Egypt
* Corresponding author. Division of Cardiology, Department of Cardiac, Thoracic and Vascular Sciences, University of Padova, Via Giustiniani 2, 35120, Padova, Italy.
E-mail address: domenico.corrado@unipd.it

in athletes.[18,19] The scope of this review is to focus on the effect of sports activity in athletes who have received an ICD for prevention of SCD, the particular problems related to ICD, and the recommendations on sports eligibility.

ICD PERFORMANCE IN ATHLETES

The accurate prediction of the performance of an ICD in athletes remains a challenging subject. Successful ICD therapy depends on a well-functioning device that is capable of appropriate sensing of the malignant arrhythmia and of delivering an adequate amount of energy to depolarize a critical myocardial mass in order to overcome the ongoing arrhythmic state. The presence of favorable myocardial physiology is paramount in achieving such critical depolarization of myocardial mass. Sports may hinder the success of ICD therapy in many aspects. First, sinus tachycardia and other supraventricular tachyarrhythmias that are often present during sports activity represent a problem for appropriate differentiation from malignant ventricular arrhythmias. Second, physiologic changes associated with exertion such as high catecholamine levels, electrolyte imbalance, metabolic acidosis, and alterations in cardiac loading can lead to arrhythmogenic states (electrical storms) whereby defibrillation may not be successful or, even worse, to SCD caused by electromechanical dissociation whereby defibrillation will not be of any benefit. Third, physical trauma, whether caused by direct or indirect contact, may lead to device injury and malfunction.

Sports Participation and ICD Interventions

There are few data concerning the relationship between sports activity and rates of ICD interventions. In 2006, Lampert and colleagues[18] conducted a survey on 614 United States Heart Rhythm Society physician members regarding the safety of sports participation in patients with ICD. With regard to the risk of shock during sports, 42% of the physicians reported that at least 1 of their patients with ICD experienced a shock during physical activity. ICD shocks were reported by 52% of physicians caring for patients competing in vigorous sports. Basketball, running, skiing (water/snow), and tennis were the most common sports associated with shocks. A second survey in Switzerland on 387 patients with ICDs reported a 14% ICD shock rate during sports activity.[20]

These studies did not assess whether the shocks reported were appropriate. Whereas appropriate therapy can be life-saving, inappropriate therapies may be dangerous and have a profound clinical and psychological impact on patients, hindering the compliance to ICD therapy.

Afterward, 2 large multicenter registry studies on children and young adult patients with ICDs demonstrated an incidence of appropriate shocks of 26% and 28%, respectively, whereas the incidence of inappropriate shocks was 21% and 25%, respectively.[21,22] Inappropriate shocks were due to triggered sinus tachycardia and supraventricular tachyarrhythmias in a rate high enough to reach the ventricular fibrillation (VF) or ventricular tachycardia (VT) detection zone. Other causes of inappropriate ICD therapy include far-field atrial activity oversensing, T-wave oversensing (**Fig. 1**),[23,24] device/lead failures (insulation failure, fracture, abrasions, or lead-pin connection failure) (**Fig. 2**),[25] and external factors leading to electromagnetic interference (transcutaneous nerve stimulation, electrocautery, and magnetic resonance equipment).[26–28]

Accurate measurements at the time of device implantation and appropriate device programming offer the potential to lower the incidence of inappropriate shocks. Both R-wave and T-wave amplitudes must be evaluated thoroughly during the implantation procedure to ensure correct sensing of the R wave without oversensing of the T wave. Several algorithms have been developed to discriminate supraventricular from VTs based on assessment of the variability of cycle length, slope of rate acceleration, and QRS duration during tachycardia (**Table 1**). A dual-chamber ICD offers the best discrimination by comparing atrial and ventricular channel rates to detect dissociation. It is important to carefully evaluate whether an upgrading of a single-chamber to a double-chamber ICD is justified for better arrhythmia discrimination, particularly in young athletes for whom conventional wisdom dictates that the fewer leads implanted, the lower the risk of lead failure and the need for extraction procedures later in life.[29]

Recently, the MADIT-RIT trial (Multicenter Automatic Defibrillator Implantation Trial—Reduce Inappropriate Therapy) showed that a significant lowering of inappropriate therapy rates was achieved by increasing the VT/VF detection rate by at least 200 beats/min or by delaying ICD intervention (with a 60-second delay at 170–199 beats/min, a 12-second delay at 200–249 beats/min, and a 2.5-second delay at ≥250 beats/min) compared with conventional programming. In this study the decrease of inappropriate therapies was associated with a trend toward mortality reduction.[30]

Sympathetic Effect on ICD Efficacy

There are conflicting findings concerning the effect of catecholamines on the efficacy of defibrillation

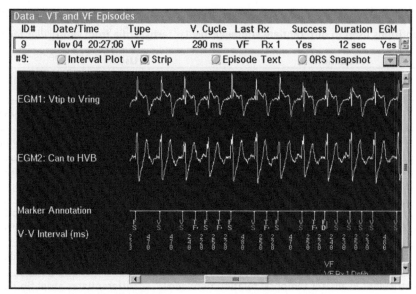

Fig. 1. Intracardiac electrogram of an implantable cardioverter-defibrillator demonstrating a T-wave oversensing, leading to double counting of the cardiac beats.

in terminating arrhythmias. Sousa and colleagues[31] demonstrated that infusion of epinephrine at dose mimicking adrenergic stimulation during mild to moderate exercise was associated with a minimal increase in defibrillation thresholds (DFTs) and a decrease in first-shock efficacy in terminating VF in ICD patients undergoing DFT testing. This observation is in agreement with the study of Venditti and colleagues[32] showing that DFT tends to be higher and first-shock efficacy lower in the morning, when the level of catecholamines is highest. On the other hand, there is emerging evidence that an ICD successfully prevents SCD during exertion. A

study on 132 patients with hypertrophic cardiomyopathy (HCM) (mean age, 34 ± 17 years, 33% younger than 20 years) by Begley and colleagues[33] found that 12% of the patients received successful appropriate ICD interventions during sports activity, proving that ICD efficacy is maintained during exercise.

Sports Injuries to the ICD System

Athletes with ICDs have an increased risk of injuring their devices, especially when engaged with sports with significant body contact. The ICD system can

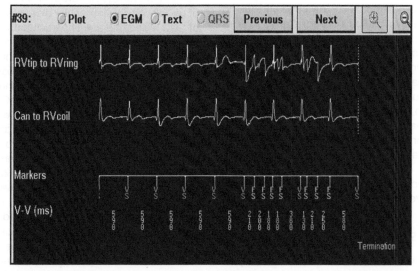

Fig. 2. Intracardiac electrogram of an implantable cardioverter-defibrillator demonstrating ventricular channel oversensing caused by lead fracture.

Table 1
Various algorithms used to differentiate supraventricular tachycardia from ventricular tachycardia

Parameter	Function	Use
Stability	Suppresses therapy for tachyarrhythmia with variable ventricular response	Differentiates atrial fibrillation
Onset	Suppresses therapy for tachyarrhythmia that slowly accelerates	Differentiates sinus tachycardia
Ventricular EGM width	Suppresses therapy for tachyarrhythmia with narrow ventricular EGM	Differentiates narrow complex SVT
Ventricular EGM morphology	Suppresses therapy for tachyarrhythmia with ventricular EGM similar to normal sinus rhythm	Differentiates narrow and wide complex SVT
Sustained rate duration	Therapy for tachyarrhythmia finally delivered after this interval	Prevents indefinite inhibition of therapy for ventricular tachycardia misdiagnosed as SVT
Atrial to ventricular ratio	Compares atrial with ventricular rate, to detect dissociation	Differentiates atrial fibrillation
Atrial to ventricular timing	Evaluates temporal relation between atrial and ventricular timing	Differentiates atrial fibrillation, 1:1 SVT retrograde conduction

Abbreviations: EGM, electrogram; SVT, supraventricular tachycardia.

be damaged, either directly as a result of blunt physical trauma, or indirectly because of repetitive bending or stretching of leads. As a consequence of electromechanical noise, the ICD device may deliver an inappropriate discharge which, in turn, may induce life-threatening ventricular tachyarrhythmias. Moreover, a damaged ICD may fail to deliver enough energy to terminate a malignant arrhythmia, for instance because of a lead break or a generator failure.

It is noteworthy that in the 2006 survey by Lampert and colleagues,[18] damage to the generator or leads was reported by only 5% of the interviewed physicians. Lead fracture or dislodgment due to indirect repetitive motion caused almost 75% of ICD-system damage, with weightlifting and golf being the most common associated sports. Direct trauma leading to generator damage was observed in just one patient during a softball game.

Another survey assessed the durability of cardiac devices with respect to sports and leisure activity in 10,000 patients younger than 21 years. Both abdominal and pectoral implants, as well as epicardial and transvenous systems, were included. Damage to devices was very uncommon (<1% per year) and is most frequently related to contact and repetitive-use sports, such as wrestling.[34]

CARDIOVASCULAR DISEASES AND SPORTS

Although arrhythmic SCD can be prevented by an ICD, participation in sports programs may be deleterious in young individuals affected by cardiac disease because systematic training may accelerate the disease progression and worsen the arrhythmic substrate. In addition, a fast VT in ICD carriers may cause syncope, which represents a potential hazard for the athlete and other competitors. These considerations go beyond the technical issues described in the previous section and further limit the sports eligibility of patients with an ICD.

Sports and Disease Progression

The most common mechanism of SCD in young competitive athletes is abrupt VF as a consequence of underlying cardiovascular diseases. The causes of SCD reflect the age of participants. Atherosclerotic coronary artery disease is the most common cause of mortality in athletes older than 35 years. In the younger athletes there is a broad spectrum of cardiovascular substrates, including congenital and inherited heart disorders (**Box 1**). Cardiomyopathies have been consistently implicated as the leading cause of sports-related cardiac arrest in the young, with HCM accounting for more than one-third of fatal cases in the United States[35,36] and arrhythmogenic right ventricular cardiomyopathy (ARVC) for approximately one-fourth of deaths in Italy.[37,38]

Corrado and colleagues[15] reported that sports activity in adolescents and young adults is associated with an increased risk of SCD. These investigators concluded that sport, per se, was not a cause of the enhanced mortality, but triggered SCD in those athletes who were affected by cardiovascular conditions predisposing to life-threatening ventricular arrhythmias during physical exercise. Arrhythmic SCD during sports usually occurs as a result of the interaction between acute external triggers, with the underlying cardiac pathology as a substrate. Extrinsic triggers during competitive sports include emotional stress, myocardial ischemia, sympathetic-vagal imbalance, and hemodynamic changes, all factors that may precipitate lethal ventricular arrhythmias.[39] On the other hand, systematic and intensive athletic training itself may increase the risk of SCD in the presence of heart disease by accelerating the progression of the underlying pathologic condition and worsening the arrhythmogenic substrate. This risk is of particular importance in young athletes carrying an ICD, as most of them suffer a genetically determined disease that tends to progress over the time. Athletes with HCM are exposed to recurrent attacks of small-vessel disease–related myocardial ischemia during intense training, with cumulative myocardial damage and fibrosis leading to ventricular electrical instability.[40] In patients with ARVC, mechanical stress linked to sustained training can accelerate myocardial fibrofatty replacement by favoring myocyte disruption and necrosis at genetically defective intercalated discs.[41]

Although there is no risk of structural disease progression in patients with cardiac ion channelopathies, sports activity and training may enhance ventricular electrical instability and increase the rate of ICD therapy. Physical exertion is the main trigger for events in patients with catecholaminergic polymorphic VT and long-QT syndrome (LQT1).[42] In patients with Brugada syndrome, malignant ventricular arrhythmias are vagally dependent and characteristically occur at rest, especially during sleep.[43] Therefore, acute sympathetic stimulation and catecholamine exposure during effort are expected to exert an inhibitory effect on the arrhythmogenic mechanisms; however, systematic conditioning in Brugada syndrome does enhance the resting vagal tone and exaggerates the vagal rebound after exercise, thus increasing the risk the occurrence of syncope or sudden death at rest or immediately after sports activity.[39]

Arrhythmic Syncope

Individuals with cardiomyopathies/channelopathies are at risk of syncope attributable to malignant ventricular arrhythmias. Latency of interrupting such tachyarrhythmias with an ICD may not prevent such syncopal attacks from happening. Syncopal events can be hazardous in certain sports where athletes may harm themselves, such as running, weightlifting, and gymnastics, or harm themselves as well as other competitors; such as canoeing and car, bicycle, or motorcycle racing. Therefore, the risk of syncope must be thoroughly evaluated before allowing an individual with an ICD to participate in such sports.[44]

SPORTS RECOMMENDATIONS AND CONTROVERSIES
Recommendations

Major American and European recommendations concerning athletes with ICDs have agreed that ICD disqualifies an athlete for competitive sports, except those with a low cardiovascular demand that do not pose a risk of trauma to the device and do not specifically trigger malignant VTs (such as torsades de pointes in congenital long-QT syndrome and polymorphic catecholaminergic VT). Sports participation can be allowed at least 6 months after the ICD implantation, or after the most recent arrhythmic episode requiring defibrillator intervention (including pacing, antitachycardia pacing, or shock). On the other hand, recommendations state that physicians and patients may feel more assured to continue leisure-time physical activities with low to moderate dynamic or static demand if an ICD is on board, which may contribute to physical and psychological well-being.[16,17,39,45]

Controversies Regarding Recommendations

Supporters of current recommendations emphasize the importance of being prudent while predicting and estimating the performance of an ICD under extreme conditions that a competitive sportsman may face, and also give prominence to differentiating between competitive and noncompetitive sports activity when implementing the restrictive recommendations. This prudent position stems from the ethical responsibility to protect the young individual's life, by avoiding all possible (although arguably unpredictable) hazards for cardiac arrest such as, in the case of patients with ICD, competitive participation in sport.[46] On the other hand, opponents of the strict recommendations argue that although there are ample theoretical reasons to restrict athletes with ICDs from sports participation, in practice, data actually proving sports to be dangerous for all ICDs and showing that competition increases the health risks in participants are nonexistent. Restricting or prohibiting competitive sports for certain patients with ICDs may develop deep psychological, physical, and financial consequences that outweigh the potential theoretical risk of harm.[19]

Recently, in an attempt to systemically assess the real-life risk in competitive sports, Lampert and colleagues[47] reported in the late-breaking trials session in Heart Rhythm 2012 the results of their prospective multinational registry on safety of sports for patients with ICDs. There were no occurrences of death or resuscitated arrest, or arrhythmia or shock-related injury during sports, and long-term freedom from lead malfunction was 90%. The investigators concluded that ICD patients should not be restricted in participating in sports because ICD therapy during athletic activity is safe.

SUMMARY

A variety of issues can limit the efficacy of ICD therapy in athletes; however, advancements in ICD manufacturing designs and programming may overcome such limitations. Looking at the bigger picture, the reasons for restriction of competitive sports in young competitive athletes with ICDs go beyond the increased risk of arrhythmias, inappropriate interventions, injury to the patient, and damage to the ICD system. Sports participation is a "mortality issue" because it plays a major role in disease progression, substrate worsening, and adverse outcome. Therefore, it is prudent to restrict participation in competitive sports for patients with ICDs. Further studies are still needed to address the risks, safety, and benefits of sports activity alongside ICD therapy.

REFERENCES

1. Mirowski M, Reid PR, Mower MM, et al. Termination of malignant ventricular arrhythmias with an implanted automatic defibrillator in human beings. N Engl J Med 1980;303:322–4.

2. The Antiarrhythmic versus Implantable Defibrillators (AVID) Investigators. A comparison of antiarrhythmic-drug therapy with implantable defibrillators in patients resuscitated from near-fatal ventricular arrhythmias. N Engl J Med 1997;337:1576–83.

3. Connolly SJ, Gent M, Roberts RS, et al. Canadian Implantable Defibrillator Study (CIDS): a randomized trial of the implantable cardioverter defibrillator against amiodarone. Circulation 2000;101:1297–302.

4. Kuck KH, Cappato R, Siebels J, et al. Randomized comparison of antiarrhythmic drug therapy with implantable defibrillators in patients resuscitated from cardiac arrest: the Cardiac Arrest Study Hamburg (CASH). Circulation 2000;102:748–54.

5. Moss AJ, Hall WJ, Cannom DS, et al. Improved survival with an implanted defibrillator in patients with coronary disease at high risk for ventricular arrhythmia. Multicenter Automatic Defibrillator Implantation Trial Investigators. N Engl J Med 1996;335:1933–40.

6. Buxton AE, Lee KL, Fisher JD, et al. A randomized study of the prevention of sudden death in patients with coronary artery disease. Multicenter Unsustained Tachycardia Trial Investigators. N Engl J Med 1999;341:1882–90.

7. Moss AJ, Zareba W, Hall WJ, et al. Prophylactic implantation of a defibrillator in patients with myocardial infarction and reduced ejection fraction. N Engl J Med 2002;346:877–83.

8. Schinkel AF, Vriesendorp PA, Sijbrands EJ, et al. Outcome and complications after implantable cardioverter defibrillator therapy in hypertrophic cardiomyopathy: systematic review and meta-analysis. Circ Heart Fail 2012;5:552–9.

9. Corrado D, Leoni L, Link MS, et al. Implantable cardioverter-defibrillator therapy for prevention of sudden death in patients with arrhythmogenic right ventricular cardiomyopathy/dysplasia. Circulation 2003;108:3084–91.

10. Corrado D, Calkins H, Link MS, et al. Prophylactic implantable defibrillator in patients with arrhythmogenic right ventricular cardiomyopathy/dysplasia and no prior ventricular fibrillation or sustained ventricular tachycardia. Circulation 2010;122:1144–52.

11. McMurray JJ, Adamopoulos S, Anker SD, et al. ESC guidelines for the diagnosis and treatment of acute and chronic heart failure 2012: the Task Force for the Diagnosis and Treatment of Acute and Chronic Heart Failure 2012 of the European Society of Cardiology. Eur J Heart Fail 2012;14:803–69.

12. Blair SN, Kohl HW, Paffenbarger RS, et al. Physical fitness and all-cause mortality. A prospective study of healthy men and women. JAMA 1989;262:2395–401.

13. Kodama S, Saito K, Tanaka S, et al. Cardiorespiratory fitness as a quantitative predictor of all-cause mortality

and cardiovascular events in healthy men and women: a meta-analysis. JAMA 2009;301:2024–35.

14. Hassmén P, Koivula N, Uutela A. Physical exercise and psychological well-being: a population study in Finland. Prev Med 2000;30:17–25.

15. Corrado D, Basso C, Rizzoli G, et al. Does sports activity enhance the risk of sudden death in adolescents and young adults? J Am Coll Cardiol 2003;42:1959–63.

16. Zipes DP, Ackerman MJ, Estes NA, et al. Task Force 7: arrhythmias. J Am Coll Cardiol 2005;45:1354–63.

17. Pelliccia A, Fagard R, Bjørnstad HH, et al. Recommendations for competitive sports participation in athletes with cardiovascular disease: a consensus document from the Study Group of Sports Cardiology of the Working Group of Cardiac Rehabilitation and Exercise Physiology and the Working Group of Myocardial and Pericardial Diseases of the European Society of Cardiology. Eur Heart J 2005;26(14):1422–45.

18. Lampert R, Cannom D, Olshansky B. Safety of sports participation in patients with implantable cardioverter defibrillators: a survey of heart rhythm society members. J Cardiovasc Electrophysiol 2006;17:11–5.

19. Lampert R, Cannom D. Sports participation for athletes with implantable cardioverter-defibrillators should be an individualized risk-benefit decision. Heart Rhythm 2008;5:861–3.

20. Kobza R, Duru F, Erne P. Leisure-time activities of patients with ICDs: findings of a survey with respect to sports activity, high altitude stays, and driving patterns. Pacing Clin Electrophysiol 2008;3:845–9.

21. Berul CI, Van Hare GF, Kertesz NJ, et al. Results of a multicenter retrospective implantable cardioverter-defibrillator registry of pediatric and congenital heart disease patients. J Am Coll Cardiol 2008;51:1685–91.

22. Von Bergen NH, Atkins DL, Dick M, et al. Multicenter study of the effectiveness of implantable cardioverter defibrillators in children and young adults with heart disease. Pediatr Cardiol 2011;32:399–405.

23. Vijayaraman P, Ferrell MS, Rhee B, et al. Implantable cardioverter defibrillator oversensing: what is the mechanism? J Cardiovasc Electrophysiol 2004;15:723–4.

24. Schimpf R, Wolpert C, Bianchi F, et al. Congenital short QT syndrome and implantable cardioverter defibrillator treatment: inherent risk for inappropriate shock delivery. J Cardiovasc Electrophysiol 2003;14:1273–7.

25. Kleemann T, Hochadel M, Strauss M, et al. Comparison between atrial fibrillation-triggered implantable cardioverter-defibrillator (ICD) shocks and inappropriate shocks caused by lead failure: different impact on prognosis in clinical practice. J Cardiovasc Electrophysiol 2012;23:735–40.

26. Casavant D, Haffajee C, Stevens S, et al. Aborted implantable cardioverter defibrillator shock during facial electrosurgery. Pacing Clin Electrophysiol 1998;21:1325–6.

27. Garg A, Wadhwa M, Brown K, et al. Inappropriate implantable cardioverter defibrillator discharge from sensing of external alternating current leak. J Interv Card Electrophysiol 2002;7:181–4.

28. Anfinsen OG, Berntsen RF, Aass H, et al. Implantable cardioverter defibrillator dysfunction during and after magnetic resonance imaging. Pacing Clin Electrophysiol 2002;25:1400–2.

29. Heidbüchel H. Implantable cardioverter defibrillator therapy in athletes. Cardiol Clin 2007;25:467–82, vii.

30. Moss AJ, Schuger C, Beck CA, et al. Reduction in inappropriate therapy and mortality through ICD programming. N Engl J Med 2012;367(24):2275–83.

31. Sousa J, Kou W, Calkins H, et al. Effect of epinephrine on the efficacy of the internal cardioverter-defibrillator. Am J Cardiol 1992;69:509–12.

32. Venditti FJ, John RM, Hull M, et al. Circadian variation in defibrillation energy requirements. Circulation 1996;94:1607–12.

33. Begley DA, Mohiddin SA, Tripodi D, et al. Efficacy of implantable cardioverter defibrillator therapy for primary and secondary prevention of sudden cardiac death in hypertrophic cardiomyopathy. Pacing Clin Electrophysiol 2003;26:1887–96.

34. Gajewski KK, Reed JH, Pilcher TA, et al. Activity recommendations in paced pediatric patients: wide variations among practitioners. Heart Rhythm 2008;5:95.

35. Maron BJ. Sudden death in young athletes. N Engl J Med 2003;349:1064–75.

36. Maron BJ, Doerer JJ, Haas TS, et al. Sudden deaths in young competitive athletes: analysis of 1866 deaths in the United States, 1980-2006. Circulation 2009;119:1085–92.

37. Corrado D, Thiene G, Nava A, et al. Sudden death in young competitive athletes: clinicopathologic correlations in 22 cases. Am J Med 1990;89:588–96.

38. Corrado D, Basso C, Thiene G. Essay: sudden death in young athletes. Lancet 2005;366(Suppl):S47–8.

39. Maron BJ, Chaitman BR, Ackerman MJ, et al. Recommendations for physical activity and recreational sports participation for young patients with genetic cardiovascular diseases. Circulation 2004;109:2807–16.

40. Basso C, Thiene G, Corrado D, et al. Hypertrophic cardiomyopathy and sudden death in the young: pathologic evidence of myocardial ischemia. Hum Pathol 2000;31:988–98.

41. Corrado D, Basso C, Thiene G, et al. Spectrum of clinicopathologic manifestations of arrhythmogenic right ventricular cardiomyopathy/dysplasia: a multicenter study. J Am Coll Cardiol 1997;30:1512–20.

42. Priori SG, Schwartz PJ, Napolitano C, et al. Risk stratification in the long-QT syndrome. N Engl J Med 2003;348(19):1866–74.

43. Matsuo K, Kurita T, Inagaki M, et al. The circadian pattern of the development of ventricular fibrillation in patients with Brugada syndrome. Eur Heart J 1999;20:465–70.

44. Law IH, Shannon K. Implantable cardioverter-defibrillators and the young athlete: can the two coexist? Pediatr Cardiol 2012;33:387–93.

45. Heidbüchel H, Corrado D, Biffi A, et al. Recommendations for participation in leisure-time physical activity and competitive sports of patients with arrhythmias and potentially arrhythmogenic conditions. Part II: ventricular arrhythmias, channelopathies and implantable defibrillators. Eur J Cardiovasc Prev Rehabil 2006;13:676–86.

46. Maron BJ, Zipes DP. It is not prudent to allow all athletes with implantable-cardioverter defibrillators to participate in all sports. Heart Rhythm 2008;5: 864–6.

47. Lampert R, Olshansky B, Heidbuchel, et al. Safety of sports for patients with ICDs: results of a prospective multinational registry. Late-breaking abstract session. Heart Rhythm 33rd Annual Scientific Sessions May 9-12, 2012, Boston.

Index

Note: Page numbers of article titles are in **boldface** type.

cardiacEP.theclinics.com

Printed and bound by CPI Group (UK) Ltd, Croydon, CR0 4YY

03/10/2024

01040346-0010